How to Get
Pregnant

Even When You've Tried Everything

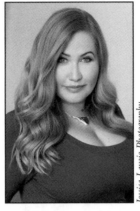

About the Author

A'ndrea Reiter is a Holistic Fertility Expert, Reiki Master, and author specializing in a mind-body approach to fertility. She uses a combination of reiki, intuition, and mindset coaching to move her clients through the emotional and physical blocks that are impeding them from conceiving naturally. Though based in Los Angeles, A'ndrea's noninvasive approach helps women all over the world to be empowered and to take charge of their fertility journeys, creating the life they want. To learn more about working with A'ndrea, visit www.FusionFertility.com.

To Write to the Author

If you wish to contact the author or would like more information about this book, please write to the author in care of Llewellyn Worldwide, and we will forward your request. Both the author and the publisher appreciate hearing from you and learning of your enjoyment of this book and how it has helped you. Llewellyn Worldwide cannot guarantee that every letter written to the author can be answered, but all will be forwarded. Please write to:

A'ndrea Reiter
⁒ Llewellyn Worldwide
2143 Wooddale Drive
Woodbury, MN 55125-2989

Please enclose a self-addressed stamped envelope for reply,
or $1.00 to cover costs. If outside the USA, enclose
an international postal reply coupon.

How to Get Pregnant

Even When You've Tried Everything

A Mind–Body Guide *to* Fertility

A'ndrea Reiter

Llewellyn Worldwide
Woodbury, Minnesota

First Edition
First Printing, 2018

Book design by Bob Gaul
Cover design by Shira Atakpu
Interior chakra figure by Mary Ann Zapalac

Llewellyn Publications is a registered trademark of Llewellyn Worldwide Ltd.

Library of Congress Cataloging-in-Publication Data
Names: Reiter, A'ndrea, author.
Title: How to get pregnant, even when you've tried everything : a mind-body
    guide to fertility / by A'ndrea Reiter.
Description: First edition. | Woodbury, Minnesota : Llewellyn Worldwide,
    [2018] | Includes bibliographical references and index.
Identifiers: LCCN 2018010483 (print) | LCCN 2018012747 (ebook) | ISBN
    9780738757223 (ebook) | ISBN 9780738756967 (alk. paper)
Subjects: LCSH: Pregnancy—Psychological aspects—Popular works. |
    Childbirth—Psychological aspects—Popular works. | Mind and body—Popular
    works.
Classification: LCC RG560 (ebook) | LCC RG560 .R45 2018 (print) | DDC
    618.2—dc23
LC record available at https://lccn.loc.gov/2018010483

Llewellyn Worldwide Ltd. does not participate in, endorse, or have any authority or responsibility
concerning private business transactions between our authors and the public.

All mail addressed to the author is forwarded, but the publisher cannot, unless specifically
instructed by the author, give out an address or phone number.

Any internet references contained in this work are current at publication time, but the publisher cannot guarantee that a specific location will continue to be maintained. Please refer to
the publisher's website for links to authors' websites and other sources.

Llewellyn Publications
A Division of Llewellyn Worldwide Ltd.
2143 Wooddale Drive
Woodbury, MN 55125-2989
www.llewellyn.com

Printed in the United States of America

Disclaimer

All information in this book is based on the author's experience and the experiences of her clients. It is shared with the understanding that you must accept responsibility for your own health. The author is not a psychologist, psychotherapist, or doctor. She will not be diagnosing you or prescribing medication, and is not advocating the foregoing of any current treatment you are receiving. Neither the author nor the publisher are legally responsible for any decisions you make based on reading this book. The purpose of this book is to make you aware of where you're putting your energy and to give you techniques to move forward through your emotional blocks. You understand that reading this book does not guarantee that you will become pregnant.

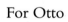

For Otto

Contents

Introduction

One in six couples have a hard time conceiving. One in six. That's approximately 7.5 to 12 million people in the United States alone. There are many reasons why. What I've found through my work in my holistic fertility practice is that often it's not for the reasons the doctors tell you.

I wrote this book because I discovered a grossly under-explored area of infertility. Some of the topics I cover are going to be new concepts to you. Some may even push your buttons. Trust me, this is good. Whenever we are getting triggered by something, it's because it is magnifying an unhealed part of ourselves—often a part that we don't want to look at. And that can be painful and can elicit some frustrating emotions. My wish is for you to use this as an opportunity to examine what's being presented and to move beyond these patterns that have been keeping you stuck. Unfortunately, sometimes that means looking at some of the things we've pushed down, things that have hurt us or things we didn't think were related to our having a baby. My request is that you take a deep breath and consider what I'm presenting. I didn't believe some of these concepts myself until I started seeing them work in my life and in my practice. And as a bonus, not only do these concepts and techniques affect fertility, but their effects ripple out to every area of your life!

I kept encountering smart, driven women who had been on excruciating journeys filled with frustration, anger, and sadness. They were making themselves crazy trying to eat the exact amount of the correct food, having sex at precisely the right moment, fearing another miscarriage, doing a fertility dance, and spending tens of thousands of dollars on invasive treatments ... and none of it was working. It broke my heart to see women who would make amazing mothers unable to get what they wanted and deserved.

But guess what? None of it has to be that way. We all hear about these women who struggled for years and then "miraculously" got pregnant. These victories don't have to be few and far between, and they don't have to happen to "other" people.

I had been working with patients dealing with chronic pain and cancer, gently introducing the idea to them that there is always an emotional cause that precipitates physical pain or health problems. Once that emotional cause is addressed, the physical condition no longer needs to be present trying to grab your attention. And my clients had some great successes.

Then I began to realize that a number of close family members and friends were having difficulty getting pregnant. They were trying everything they'd been told to do, but it wasn't working. I thought, well, the same principles should apply to fertility that apply to other physical conditions, so I began working with my sister-in-law. She'd had two losses and wasn't sure she even wanted to try again. But in six months she was pregnant, and nine months later my little nephew debuted on the planet. This spurred me to begin empowering as many women as possible to take charge of their journeys, and it's been the most fulfilling thing I've ever done.

I work with my private clients using a combination of reiki (to clear energy blocks and heal physical and emotional issues), intuition (tapping into my client's subconscious to see what experiences and beliefs are holding her back), and mindset coaching (techniques that help my clients process and release whatever traumas or beliefs have been unearthed). This three-pronged approach is key in moving women through their blocks. The mindset component is *the* thing that makes the difference in whether or not they are getting pregnant. It's absolutely paramount that you learn to retrain your brain and rewire your thought process. When you do, things begin to shift on a cellular level, and so-called miracles happen.

This book will help you see that you can create your own "miracle." You have *way* more power on this fertility journey than you've been led to believe. This knowledge can help you get more connected to your intuition and your body as opposed to your head. Unfortunately we have drifted further and further from our connection with our bodies. So we rely on doctors and other well-meaning people to tell us what's wrong with us. We are subconsciously affected by the fear-mongering and insensitivity that strip us of our innate power.

Did you know that in many European countries it's not unheard of for a woman to have a healthy baby at fifty years old? Why, in the US, are they warning us that our biological clock is ticking out at twenty-eight? Entertain the idea that our capability to conceive doesn't necessarily just drop severely on its own, but rather it might be due to a combination of factors we don't even realize are operating in the background. The awesome thing is that they're all *changeable*! Consider the possibility that this journey doesn't have to be horrible. That your body isn't failing you. That you have the power to shift your situation.

I am so grateful for all of my clients who've helped me learn as much as I've helped them to grow. You are warriors. You are rock stars. You are my heroes. Thank you for being brave and for being open to taking the reins of your journey.

This book is presented in six chapters and outlines the areas where we can get stuck and how we can move forward. It was purposely written as a "girlfriend's guide." It is intentionally not medical or cold or sterile. I'm writing to you as if you were my best friend and private client. We will be looking at external factors affecting fertility, beliefs, physical conditions, and the Law of Attraction as it applies to fertility. They are really all so interconnected that it's hard to separate them. But hopefully this gives you an idea of why and how we want to start shifting our thoughts so we can literally change our physical conditions and our *life*.

To gain the greatest value from this book, I invite you to visit my website, www.FusionFertility.com, and register to receive your free Conceivable Tool Kit. Inside you will find tips and exercises to guide you along your fertility journey. All the worksheets referenced in this book are included in the tool kit.

So take a deep breath, keep an open mind, and dive in. You can do this. And I'm excited to show you how.

Lots of love,
A'ndrea

1

....

External Factors

The outside influences that can mess with your fertility

We're going to cover a lot about energy and mindset in this book, but first we'll talk about the fifteen external factors that could be affecting your fertility. These are outside factors that might not immediately seem related to your fertility but can be huge contributing factors. Obviously not everyone who has these factors deals with infertility, but this is where the mindset and the external factor together can block fertility. Not all fifteen will apply to you, but it's very likely that, as we elaborate on each factor, one you didn't think was an issue might resonate. Also notice if something other than these fifteen comes up for you.

I'm going to bring your awareness to things that can be affecting your fertility and ways to diminish or even eliminate these factors. I invite you to write in your own ideas on the 15 External Factors worksheet in the Conceivable Tool Kit if something comes to you.

Let's begin with the first factor on your sheet.

1. Stressful Job

While most people think their job is stressful, I'm talking mainly about teachers, nurses, caregivers, and CEOs—those responsible for groups or teams of people. You get to work early, stay late, and give it your all. You're great at your job.

But here's the problem:

Your brain/ego's main function is to keep you alive. The amygdalae in your brain are two almond-shaped groups of nuclei located in the temporal lobes. They play a primary role in memory, decision-making, and emotional reactions. This is where aggression, addiction, anxiety, PTSD, and, most importantly, fear reside. The amygdalae are responsible for the primal fight-or-flight reflex. This response is awesome when you're being chased by wolves, but not so much when you're trying something new. Your brain means well and wants to keep you safe, but sometimes it's a pain in the ass. While we don't live in a world where we need to run from saber-toothed tigers anymore, our brain is still triggered by stressors that it perceives as a threat to our survival. When we have too many things going on and are spread too thin, it triggers a silent alarm in our body. That's when things can start to go haywire. The fight-or-flight response is part of the sympathetic nervous system, which means it's automatic; and it can be triggered on a low-grade level without our even realizing it sometimes.

When you're responsible for a lot of people's health and wellbeing, such as a teacher, nurse, or caregiver, or you're responsible for a team in a corporate situation, your time and energy are maxed out. So while *you're* thinking "I want to have a baby," your brain already feels as though it's taking care of way too many people and says, "Why would we add another responsibility to our plate?" It *literally* can't handle taking care of another human, and that can put the kibosh on the lady parts.

When you're in fight-or-flight mode, all unnecessary body systems slow or shut down. All available energy goes to the heart, brain, lungs, and legs (in case of flight). During a crisis, you don't need your reproductive system to stay alive. This is especially prevalent among women in the unexplained infertility group. When the doctor can't find anything wrong with you, this very thing could be happening. Though it may seem like only low-grade stress to you, it's not to your body. This continual stress pattern, over a long period of time, is exhausting. Again, not everyone in these careers has fertility issues, but 95 percent of my clients are in these fields. There's an undeniable correlation.

So what can we do about it?

You might say, "Okay, great, but I can't quit my job right now," or "I love my job. Am I screwed?"

Of course not.

Are you the get-there-early-and-leave-late, give-it-your-all type? While that's admirable and will garner you perks at work, this push-to-the-limit attitude could actually be getting in the way of conceiving. Your great work ethic is awesome, but unfortunately it can mean you're taking care of everyone else's needs before your own. So your lovely brain, which wants to keep you alive, says, "Um, we're already stretched way too thin and not taking care of ourselves as it is. And you want to *add* something to our plate? Are you *insane*?!" I'm certainly not advocating that you become a sloth and only move for food and sex, but we do want to look at ways you can slowly start conserving more energy. When your brain feels that you have more space in your life, the fight-or-flight response isn't triggered as often, and it will feel that a baby is a plausible venture.

Even though you, as an evolved human, want the baby and see all the positives, you are dealing with a primal, involuntary reaction in the brain that you cannot fool. So our initial job is to create an environment where your brain feels safe to start this process.

Consider it food for thought that when most of my clients come to me for fertility assistance, they also end up changing their career in some capacity. So I invite you to inquire in a journal entry if you're in the career you feel you're *meant* to be in, or one you feel you're *obligated* to be in. More and more I'm seeing these two areas tied together, and sometimes it can be the reason the baby hasn't shown up yet. You're supposed to get a handle on that first.

When we want to have a baby so badly, we tend to skip over the areas where we need to do some work or make adjustments. But that work, ladies, is what helps you move toward the baby. These roadblocks being presented to you are not to be jumped over or gone around. You must move through them. They are likely a big part of why your pregnancy hasn't happened yet. In your career, you need confidence, drive, preparedness, and the feeling of being capable.

More often than not, my clients tend to be in a job that is just that … a job. It's a paycheck, or it gives them professional accolades, but it doesn't feed their soul. I'll ask them, "What do you want to be when you grow up?" I've only had one person answer that it was what they were currently doing. On the surface that might not seem important, but I'm finding that we are being called to step into our *purpose* versus a career. When we are not in that purpose—the reason we are on the planet this time around—other things that we really want can be delayed. That delay is not your body failing you; it's trying to give you time to find your purpose before you add another aspect to your life.

I have my clients explore what they'd love to do for a living if their "stories" about why they couldn't do it didn't factor in. I joke that if they want to be a mime in a park, we'll find a way to make it happen. But seriously, if you're harboring a super-creative person buried under an overworked CPA, it could be a problem. There's nothing wrong with being a CPA if that's your purpose, but if your soul longing isn't being fed, it can manifest in your body. I'll get more into chakras later in the book, but for now know that there are seven main wheels of energy in your body, going from the base of your spine to the top of your head. They all represent something different.

When I'm reading people, the sacral chakra, located at your lower abdomen, represents creativity, relationships, and children. Your ovaries and uterus quite literally represent the point of creation. So if you are in a job that's not feeding your soul, feeding your creativity, that chakra can be closed. That means the creating children part shuts down as well. I'm not saying quit your job and draw landscapes on the sidewalk with chalk; but finding a way to feed your soul, whether it's with something obviously creative (painting, drawing, dancing, photography) or something that just feeds your passion (getting a yoga teacher certification, making organic bath products, flipping houses) is a key component in how fast you move forward. Stepping out of the idea of being obligated to be in a job and into what were you put on the planet to do is so important.

Here are some things you can implement now to convince your brain there's room for a baby:

- If you usually stay late at work, commit to staying late only two days a week this month, then only one day a week the next month. If you can, wean over time to zero. But even if you stay at one, that's a hell of a lot better than five.

- If you are on one or more committees/organizations at work, cut down your involvement or pass it on to someone else and stop completely. Two of my clients who are teachers were involved in several extra things besides their teaching responsibilities, such as teachers union committee, AP classes, tutoring, department head, taking master's classes, and club advisors. These are *all* admirable things, but they're little things that add up to a lot of your energy. Again, if your brain feels overloaded with all that you have to do for so many other people, it believes that it literally can't take on anything else. Can you find a place to back off on some of these responsibilities? Ask yourself, "If I had to choose between one of these extra things and my baby, would I still choose to be head of my union?" The mistake a lot of women make is thinking, "When I get pregnant I'll cut back." But the overload could be the *very* thing preventing you from getting pregnant, so take that action now. Put out to the Universe that you're making space for this munchkin to show up. In chapter 4, we will get into why that energy is so important.

- Show the Universe that you're energetically choosing
  the baby. Find ten minutes a day (and yes, you have it) to
  implement some sort of grounding practice. It's all right if
  you're not into yoga or meditation, though that'd be great.
  Having this daily practice, even if it's for only a few minutes a
  day, starts to train the brain that you're safe, you're taking care
  of yourself, and it's okay to allow this baby in.
  You can do something as simple as

  - taking a bath with essential oils.

  - sitting in the park or near a patch of grass on your
    lunch break and connecting to the earth.

  - listening to soothing music with your hand on your
    belly, inviting in the baby's energy.

  - having a solo dance party in your living room to
    "Eye of the Tiger," Lady Gaga, or whatever floats your
    fertility boat. The idea is to get you into your body and
    out of your head.

If your schedule is maxed out, you must find a way to create
space so that your brain can feel like there's room for this baby
to come in.

2. Family Pressure

Many of us, from the moment we're married, are asked, "When are you
having kids?" Parents are eager for a grandchild to spoil. We're also so
steeped in tradition as a society that it's just what you do. You have a baby
after you get married. We're almost trained to ask that question.

Although family and friends mean well, their comments can seem
preachy, judgy, or just plain insensitive. When we're dealing with fertility
issues, we're already feeling insecure, and the last thing our brain wants is
to feel worse about the situation. Not only are we worrying about our

own feelings, but we then take on that extra responsibility of being able to tell our friends and family some good news. We plug it into our belief system the idea that "we should be pregnant by now." The pressure of multiple people counting on us gets painful. And every time we encounter those people, we start to dread the inevitable question. We will talk more about beliefs in chapter 2, but suffice it to say that it wears on us.

Part of what keeps this pressure going is that we don't always want our family to know we're having a hard time getting pregnant. Though I hope this will change in the near future, infertility has traditionally been a very private struggle. So we think that if we share our issues, our loved ones will judge us or offer unsolicited advice that can be unintentionally painful. On the flip side, if we don't address their comments, it continues to fester in us and perpetuates the problem. Social situations that were once fun turn into a tedious, defensive chore.

First of all, there's no shame in this journey at *all*. And honestly, the more it's talked about, the better. Fertility is one of the few taboo issues left. It used to be like that with cancer and PTSD, but now they're openly talked about. Unfortunately there is still shame around infertility, because we feel our body is not doing what women's bodies have done for millennia. We blame ourselves. Remember that one in six women struggles with infertility. It's very likely that you know multiple women who've dealt with the same thing. Realizing that you are not defective is so important in this journey. Just because the check engine light comes on in the car doesn't mean the car is a lemon. Addressing the issue removes the stigma.

Many of us have that family member or friend who continually asks when we're having kids. As I said, that can be energetically draining. You put on a brave face and swallow your frustration. Every family party and dinner out with friends where you have to do this gets stored in your body—the annoyance, the frustration, the stress, the shame, the fear. Under the umbrella of the Law of Attraction is the Law of Psychophysical Response, which says that for every stressful thought, there is a stressful reaction in the body. Studies show that when we relive stressful past experiences or even hypothetical future scenarios, our bodies actually react as though it's happening now. Every time you tell someone about it or think about it, your body is stressing in real time. It's so interesting! Consider the effect that these thoughts have on your body each time someone asks you at work or the next baby shower, "So, when are *you* having kids?"

The problem with this, besides feeling annoying and hurtful, is that it's actually impacting your body. When your body is in even a low state of fight-or-flight, it's enough for your reproductive system to slow or shut down. Think about the primal fight-or-flight response: You need your heart, brain, lungs, and feet (in case of flight) to get out of a stressful situation. The last thing you need is for your reproductive system to be fully functional. So if not for your own sanity, do the following exercise for your body and your future baby.

We take on a lot of responsibility when we're worried about letting family down. It's hard enough to deal with how *you* feel. To take on someone else's expectations can be really overwhelming. Perpetuating these stressful thoughts takes a toll on the body. The good news is that according to the same law, for every positive thought you have, there is a corresponding response in your body. It's important that we choose positive thoughts and surround ourselves with positive people for this reason.

EXERCISE

My challenge to you is to say something to them, not from defensiveness, anger, or fear but from a loving place. You hopefully understand that they just want the best for you. And because they aren't going through it, they have *no idea* how it's affecting you. All they know to say is "Just relax" and "It's up to God." Know that, infuriating as that is, it's coming from a caring place. *But* that doesn't mean you should have to keep swallowing your feelings about their constant inquiries.

Speaking to them *once* about it can save numerous times of them asking. While I totally agree that it's none of their beeswax, it saves *you* a perpetual headache. Swallowing your frustration can squash your energy and ability to allow a baby in.

A lot of times, that family member or friend has their own neurosis that they're projecting onto you, and you're absorbing it without even being aware of it. For example, before she was pregnant, one of my clients (who just gave birth to twins) was dealing with pretty severe anxiety. As we worked together, we saw that her mother was projecting all her fears onto her daughter. My client was subconsciously scared of being pregnant and of life in general. We did a lot of belief work, which we'll get to in chapter 2, but to summarize here, once she realized they were her mom's fears and not hers, she was able to speak frankly to her mom and stop the IV of anxiety and get pregnant.

Some people will casually bring up the subject not knowing that it's been a struggle that you're sensitive about. Not having gone through it, they can't possibly know their nonchalant comments are actually coming across as insensitive. It could also be that friends and family members are just genuinely excited for you. They can't wait to have a little munchkin to spoil. They know you're going to be an awesome mom and can't wait for this next phase of life to start for you.

Whatever the case may be—and it may be all three in various areas of your life—there's a way you can approach it that will bring about understanding versus hurt feelings on one or both sides. It's likely that they don't know they are doing anything that's hurtful, so if you lash out, both sides are hurt. Then there's no lasting understanding, because to them it will seem like your reaction is coming out of nowhere.

On the flip side, you don't want to constantly be defending your position to a pushy family member. Everyone's got an opinion, and if yours doesn't match Aunt Susie's, it can be a little daunting. One of my clients wanted to take a more holistic route, while her mother was pushing every intervention known to man. It was mentally and energetically wearing on my client. So we talked about finding a way to come from a loving but *clear* place about what her boundaries were.

Try something to the effect of this:

"_____ , I understand that you mean well and are excited for me. I know you love me and want the best for me and/ or are just curious, so I need you to hear this. _____ and I are in the process of starting a family. I so appreciate your love and concern, but it stresses me out when people keep asking about our baby-making status. I'm really focusing on grounding and being peaceful and present right now. I love that you're excited to be a _____ (grandparent, aunt, etc.). Just know that when there's good news to report, you will be one of the first to hear. In the meantime, we are exploring all the avenues that feel right for us. Thanks for your support."

You don't want to admonish them. They're your loved ones and genuinely want to see you happy. They just don't realize how their inquiries are affecting you. Thank them for their love and concern while being clear about what you need. Remember that they aren't doing it to piss you off or make you feel less than. And by addressing them in this way, you can head off a lot of your own frustration. That's honestly the most important thing. We want to get you into a safe, supported, stress-free environment as much as possible. And heading off well-meaning friends and family at the pass can save a lot of energy.

3. Partner's Energy Is Holding Back

This factor may be seen in the following ways:

- It may physically manifest as male infertility (which we will go into more in depth in chapter 3).

- He's getting cold feet about the amount of responsibility of having a child.

- He hasn't achieved what he wants in his career yet.

- He's got some subconscious family issues going on—parents never around or father left, etc.—and he hasn't really dealt with it.

Sometimes we get so gung-ho about having a baby that we can unintentionally miss our partner's concerns and sweep them under the rug. But it doesn't solve anything and you just have a really big lump under your rug. It's important to step out of your situation and see if any of these scenarios might apply to your partner.

Even if you are willing to work with him, many husbands/partners are hesitant to consider non-medical alternatives—especially ones that have an energy component—so it can be hard to get them on board to move forward. And honestly sometimes it takes them seeing *you* making progress with this before they'll ease in, but there are things you can do to help your partner's energy move forward without going all woo-woo on them and freaking them out.

Close your eyes and take a deep breath. Visualize your partner in front of you, tune in to their energy, and ask:

- Are they in a career they hate?

- Is there still something they want to be when they grow up that I could encourage?

- Is there a class or workshop they could take to move their energy in that direction?

Most times they aren't aware of how to move through it, or sometimes they don't even know they're stuck. Sometimes supporting them and pointing them in that direction is enough to shift things.

I've seen this many times with men with low sperm count and motility. (We'll get more into that in chapter 3.) It often comes down to them not being in the career they would love, or the fact that the woman is the breadwinner or the more dominant personality.

You might know what his dream career would be, or you might not. If you don't, casually ask. Even if money and schedule are tight, what might be some ways that he could move toward it? Workshops? Classes? Meetups? If you can't think of any class or certification he could pursue, you could just do some research about his desired career in your area or encourage a hobby that fulfills him. My client Amy's husband was in a job he hated and wanted to be a firefighter. Finances wouldn't allow that at the moment, so he joined the volunteer brigade and felt more fulfilled. As a result, his sperm count and motility improved.

In another case, my client Rae was pretty high up in corporate America, and her husband made much less than she did. She also made all of the household decisions. It sounds a little silly, but men still have that primal instinct to provide. They still innately feel the need to kill the food, drag it back, and see their family live because of them. So with Rae taking care of the "hunting" and the home front, her husband was left unsure of his place and certainly not feeling like a provider. In chapter 3 we will go into how this directly affects the body, but for now know that when a man isn't feeling important or valid or that he has a primary role in the function of the family, his sperm motility and count can be affected.

Did I ask Rae to quit the prestigious position she loved, just so her husband could feel important? Of course not. There are other ways that men can feel like they're contributing, even if it's not financial. It could be something as simple as having him do a DIY project that you've been meaning to knock off the list for a while, or getting the car serviced, taking out the trash, or other things that need to be done to keep your lives running smoothly.

We want to be careful that it's not just giving chores to a kid. The important part of this is that you let him know how helpful it was that he did said task. It was such a big help, relief, took something off your plate, etc. Thanking him for making your life easier goes a long way with men. Not only are they more likely to keep doing a task when they are praised for it, but energetically they feel like they have a greater purpose, more worth, etc. That's when we can start to see changes in the morphology.

Also look at his family situation:

- Are both of his parents still in the picture?

- Are they divorced? If so, how old was he at the time of the divorce?

- Has he not fully grieved or processed the death of a parent?

- Are there abandonment issues that he doesn't want to repeat?

- Talk with him as lovingly and supportively as possible. This sounds like a no-brainer, but often when we want to be pregnant so badly, we want our partner to hurry up and figure it out so we can move forward. Look at him as the person you love the most in the world who might be a little stuck and do what you can to connect to and love him. It will trickle down to the baby, but for right now, you may have to focus on him. So open your heart and see if you can feel into how you might best be able to help him move through this block.

- If he doesn't know what the problem is or won't talk about it, see if he'll try acupuncture—so the energy can be unblocked, regardless of whether he wants to share his feelings or not. Acupuncture is a relatively accepted modality, even for men who aren't really into alternative methods.

- If you have good friends who have kids and your husband/
partner is close with the other husband, have the friend talk
to him to alleviate his fears.

All of the manifestations of male infertility come from fears and beliefs
that he's likely not even consciously aware of. So take some time away
from the stress of getting pregnant and plug yourself into lovingly helping your partner forward.

4. Is Your Relationship Solid?

Some of the aforementioned things apply here, but this is more about
the two of you. This can be a tough factor to really look at, so if this
applies to you, try to breathe into it and see how you can move forward.
When we are on Mission Baby, it's so easy to want to skip over the pesky
relationship thing.

Here's the thing: the obstacle *is* the path. That's a famous saying and
it's so true. This obstacle was put in front of you to move through—not
to leap over or burrow under or find a way around. The Universe is a
loyal friend, albeit that tough-love friend that you want to punch but
know it's right. We'll get into why this is the case energetically in chapter 4, but for now know that avoiding our blocks doesn't make them go
away. Sure, we can choose not to deal with it now, but the pattern will
keep repeating until we move through it, so why not address it and be
done with it? Yes, it can be messy and painful, but honestly that's better
than staying in some kind of weird relationship limbo. Don't hope that
getting pregnant will change your relationship. Change your relationship
so you can get pregnant. Ask yourself:

- Do you fight a lot? More than you get along?

- Does the divorce word get thrown around?

- Are you out separately with friends more than together?

- Is there physical or verbal abuse going on?

I know this seems like an unpleasant topic, but two of my clients, Jasmine and Diane, have gone through some combo of these issues and both chose very different paths. Neither is right or wrong. It's more about making a decision.

Their husbands wouldn't go to counseling because "nothing was wrong with them." Their wives were putting so much energy into the relationship and not getting anything back. They were being made to feel small and insignificant—and believe me, the worth piece does a number on fertility. If you don't feel capable in one area of your life, it's really difficult to feel capable in others.

We can't change our partners or *make* them do what we want. We can't *change* anybody. But we *can* and *must* change how we react to this challenge we are being presented with. Do we find a way to move through the obstacle and stay, or do we leave and start over? Sometimes through the belief work (in chapter 2) we are able to shift our energy and viewpoint about what's happening in the relationship and release negative energy about it and move forward. That being said, abuse is never okay and should not be tolerated. There's always a lesson to learn on an energetic level, but I am by no means condoning staying in an abusive relationship.

So often we feel like if we leave now, it's gonna take *way* too long to meet someone else, get married, get pregnant, and have a baby. We already feel like we're running out of time (which isn't true, by the way, and we'll get to that in chapter 2), so we might as well stay.

I promise you, if the relationship isn't fixed one way or the other, you're going to keep spinning your wheels.

We want a baby so badly sometimes that we're willing to leap over the relationship problem to get to the baby.

Remember that energetically, this roadblock is being put there for you to address, not to leap over.

Admittedly, that can seem like a huge pain in the ass. But see if you can look at it by asking yourself, "What do I need to learn from this first?

What is the gift I'm supposed to be getting out of this?" This can be a hard question to answer, especially if your partner doesn't know how to communicate or the relationship has been deteriorating for quite a while. I promise that there is always a reason we are going through what we are going though, and the timing isn't random. The things that happen to us aren't because of a vengeful god or because we're being punished for cheating on that spelling test in fifth grade. There are always lessons to be learned. That phrase can have a not-so-great connotation to it. When we were little and heard the phrase "I hope you learned your lesson," it usually meant we'd been punished for doing something we shouldn't have done or that shouldn't have happened. So we can be a little gun-shy when it comes to us having to learn "life lessons."

I'd like to reframe that a little bit. Whether you believe in reincarnation or not, I like to refer to our life this time around on Earth as "Earth Camp." I believe that each time around we pick things to "work on," whether it's family, relationships, health, or money. These are not easy things to move through, but if we do, we acquire skills that up-level us, so to speak; and if we don't, we repeat it the next time until we do get it. So everything we come across in this incarnation on Earth Camp is a class with something to learn. As long as we don't assign a stressful meaning to the thing, it can be as simple as taking history, algebra, or a relationship class. Yes, in some cases it's a doctoral-thesis kind of class, but it's for us to learn, not something to harm us. I like to say that it's happening *for* you, not *to* you. We will live through it, though it doesn't feel like it at the time. So the more we can say, "Okay, this sucks and is really stressful right now, but I'm in this situation to learn something, so what might that be?" There is an answer. I will bet lots and lots of money on it.

In the case of my client Jasmine, her husband was super high-strung and was always going to put work first, and he verbally abused her to keep her small. He had addictions he wouldn't deal with, and her lesson was to take back her power and believe that she could do or be anything she wanted. She moved back among her friends and family and blossomed. She found love soon after and was pregnant eight months later at forty-one! So her not getting pregnant with her former husband was a sign for her to deal with the relationship.

My client Diane had a similar experience in terms of being made to feel small—her husband was squashing her personality because she was "too much," and he was verbally abusive and unsupportive. He threatened divorce on a daily basis and told her that she was the problem and he had nothing to work on. He was also lacking in some social skills and had to deal with an overbearing mother who controlled everything well past the normal timeline. He either chose not to leave his mother's nest or wasn't allowed to, but his mother overstepped boundaries by continuing to try to make decisions for him even after he was married, and to make my client feel like a burden and less than.

Diane realized her husband hadn't learned certain things about relationships because of being sheltered by his overbearing mother. Things like how to work through disagreements without threatening divorce. That the way your wife does things isn't necessarily how your mother does them and that's okay. That once you're married, the two of you are a nuclear unit and make all decisions, financial and otherwise, together. That you don't squash the other person's personality to make it fit your ideals. My lovely client, who wanted to make this relationship work, was the more evolved of the pair and did a lot of work on herself to clean up her beliefs and blocks so that she could be in a place to help him through his and move forward as a team. She made the decision to stay and was able to get pregnant.

So whatever you decide, the important thing is that you decide something and take action in that direction. The Universe can't bring you what you want when you're in a place of limbo.

When there's another person involved in the decision, it makes it more complicated. We can't change that person and we can't make them get on board with our plan. We can't make them heal themselves or the relationship if they are not willing. So in order to assess where they are, we need to crack open our heart and tell them about our dreams for a family and for the relationship, and our desire to work on things, go to therapy, and exhaust all options before throwing in the towel, plus how much we really love and value them, etc., and then see where they are mentally. If they are willing to recognize that they need to work on things as well and are willing to do what they can to preserve the relationship, fantastic! Together you can outline some steps and a timeline for the goals of the relationship and begin moving forward. Having a heart-to-heart really helped my client Diane to stay, because she saw a different side of her husband and his commitment to implementing solutions and moving forward. We want to know that we are on the same team and that the other person has our back. So having a heart-to-heart can strip away the stories we have in our head about the other person and allow us to see them in a vulnerable state and reconnect with them. Often, by working on ourselves and bringing our energy up, they will rise up to meet us.

If your partner says you're the problem and he has nothing to work on, first of all, that's not true. I don't care if the ratio is 50-50, 70-30, or 99-1, but there is never one person who is completely at fault in an argument or a relationship. We can get ourselves so closed off because of our hurt and frustration about the other person and so plugged into our "stories" about it that it can seem like the other person is the problem. But there is always something to work on. No one's ever done or finished early. Everyone has crap to work on. Unfortunately, if your partner can't see that you both have things to work on, it can be hard to move forward. If you are funneling energy into something and not getting anything back, that can mean that it may be better for you to move on, as Jasmine did. If you are staying small, giving up your dreams, and walking on eggshells around your partner, that is not even remotely conducive to conceiving a baby. And leaving could mean that you're allowing in that next partner, like the one who came for Jasmine just months later.

Leaving didn't stop her from being a mom, and it didn't take nearly as long to have a baby as her brain thought it would.

Close your eyes and put your hand on your heart and ask yourself which scenario feels right for you. We cannot make the decision to stay or go out of fear of what our partner will do, fear of what will happen to our dream of having a baby, or fear that we will make the wrong decision. We will talk more in chapter 4 about how to align your energy with what you want versus what you don't want, but making a decision from a calm, plugged-in place will ensure that you're doing the right thing.

5. Too Cerebral (Not in Your Body)

Many women dealing with fertility issues are not connected to their bodies. They're smart women who are good at their jobs and figuring things out, but there's a disassociation from the body that can happen that can exacerbate the infertility issue. We are essentially driving our meat suit around from our head and are often disconnected from our intuition as a result.

Just as the third eye is an accepted center of intuition, so is your gut. I'm sure you've heard the term "gut feeling." But so many of us like to think and analyze things down to a bloody stump, to the point that we are completely unaware of what our intuition is trying to tell us, and we get frustrated when our body doesn't do what we want or think it should do (which we will talk about more in chapter 3). We feel that our body is failing us and that if we could just get it on board with our brilliant plan, everything would be fine. We need our body in order to have a baby, but if we are treating it like this unfortunate ball and chain that we have to drag around, it's very hard to be connected to it and to conceive.

It's also likely that if you're super-cerebral, it's not so easy for you to feel into the emotions of things. So we want to look at some ways to get you more aware of your feelings and how to direct them toward what you want, as well as to bridge the gap between your brain and body by learning to listen to your intuition. Now this may seem easier said than done. As with any habit or pattern, it takes time. But here are a couple of exercises to get you started.

EXERCISE

It's hard sometimes for us cerebral folks to just "get into our bodies." So sometimes having visual cues can help us connect to our body and therefore have more access to our intuition. Close your eyes and visualize a tiny purple elevator sitting at the top of your head. Close the door of the elevator and watch it start to descend to your forehead. Taking deep, slow breaths, see the elevator move down to your throat, down to your heart, and lowering deeper still to your upper abdomen. Your breathing slows down as the elevator descends into your lower abdomen and finally comes to a stop at the base of your spine.

Once you're dropped down into your body, place a hand on your abdomen and just ask a question, like "What do I need to know/do in order to move forward?" Now here's the tricky part: we want to not be attached to getting an answer. We will get into attachment in chapter 4, but for now, just ask the question and be open to receiving whatever comes. It may be a visual, a color, or a feeling, or you may hear a sentence. You may hear nothing for the first week of doing this. It's okay! You wouldn't expect to be able to learn and speak Aramaic in the span of a week. Cut yourself some slack and just keep calling in the energy of the next best step for you. Write down whatever you do notice, even if it seems insignificant. If you get the color blue one day and an ostrich the next, write it down. See if you can feel into what they might mean. You can also look up the symbolism of the things that come up, but I find it best to feel into what it means for you.

When developing your intuition, the hardest thing is to trust it. When I was developing mine, I remember saying more often than not, "Is that my intuition or my imagination?" While it is difficult to discern at the beginning, you need your imagination to access your intuition. This is why it's important to write everything down each time you do this. The more you do it, the more you will see patterns or coincidences, and you'll begin to trust yourself more. We will dig more into intuition in chapter 2, but it's essential that we learn how to be in our body instead of driving it around from our head. There are things that our body is trying to tell us, and the more connected we are to it, the more we can interpret the information and take action to move the mind and body forward together versus pulling them in opposite directions.

EXERCISE

Here is an exercise for getting a little more connected to your emotions. Close your eyes and think of a time when you were really sad or angry (a relationship ended, your boss was mean to you, someone passed away, etc.). Notice where in your body you feel that thought (in the pit of your stomach, wanting to vomit, wanting to give up, blood boiling, etc.). Notice what that thought does to your body.

Now wipe that visual slate clean and shake it off. Close your eyes again and imagine a time when you were really excited about something (the day your partner proposed, when you got a promotion, when you got a puppy, etc.). Notice where in your body you feel that thought (butterflies in your stomach, goose bumps/chills, can't stop smiling/laughing, etc.). Notice what that thought does to your body.

We get so caught up in our day-to-day routines that we rarely check in to see how our emotions are affecting our body, especially if we lean toward the cerebral end of the spectrum. So take some time to take stock of your emotions and see how you really *feel* about something versus what you *think* about it. We will get into this more in chapter 4, but when we feel things (versus thinking about them), that's when things begin to shift on a cellular level in the body.

It took me about two months to get my client Leah to be able to assess how she was feeling, not her thoughts about her feelings but how she *felt*. As an academic with multiple long-standing family issues, she was great at having the drive to get things done, but she had zero idea about what was going on with her emotions. Emotions seemed like a hazard or certainly a huge inconvenience to her, so it was best to be strong and not care—all the time. This started to take a toll on her physical body, which we will get into in chapter 3. Her check engine light was saying, "Hey! We need to process some shit! And since you won't look at it, it's affecting the vessel that makes the baby you want so desperately." Using the previous two exercises helped her get to a place where she could check in with how she was feeling and to process things so that she could heal her body and therefore get pregnant. Most of us are like Leah in that we don't like looking at our uncomfortable emotions. After all, who *wants* to feel anger, sadness, hopelessness? This is, however, part of the process of healing (as we will see in chapter 4) and is also important in terms of getting your body to a place where it feels positive and safe to bake this baby.

6. Super Planner/Micromanager

I say this lovingly to all my Type-A compadres: We get shit done, right? And most of the time that's a good thing, but when it comes to the arrival of our munchkin, it can be a little frustrating when it doesn't happen when we want it to. Whenever we think we can control everything, the Universe has a little laugh and says, "Oh yeah?" All of a sudden it's like, "What the hell happened to my plans?" We want to get pregnant at 7:01 p.m. on April 17 in Paris because that's when it's convenient and fantastic for us. It sounds funny, but some of us really can get like that about our timelines. We want everything to fit into this nice box, but the Universe has other ideas.

Relinquishing our need to control things is perhaps the trickiest part of this whole process. Most of us already know if we are a bit of a control freak or not. Chances are, if we are team Type A, we probably have a bit of a control issue.

Sometimes this just manifests as needing to be tidy all the time, or else we get nervous; but some women are entrenched in having to deal with a more extreme manifestation, like OCD. These can be things that have developed from a point in childhood or adulthood where we have felt an extreme loss of control and have put the manifestation of that into an action or need. It may not seem directly related to your uterus, but the fear of not having control perpetuates more fear (which keeps your fight-or-flight switch on).

EXERCISE

If you have a need to control, take a deep breath and visualize whatever your specific issue is (the load of laundry that needs to be done, the bed that needs to be made, etc.). Feel what that's like in your body. How much does it bug you? How compelled are you to finish the task? Where do you feel that in your body?

Then say, "If I didn't *need* to do the laundry or make the bed, how would I feel? If the dishwasher isn't unloaded today or I don't make the bed, what will happen? Will anyone die? Will something bad happen?" It feels like it sometimes. But we need to give ourselves a break, because maybe it's more important to take a bath or watch a movie with the hubby. See if you can zoom out of your body and look at the compulsion as just a thought. It's not a reality that you will die or anything bad will happen, it's just your brain's story about the thought.

Can you just sit in the discomfort of the thought long enough to realize nothing will happen? Then, don't make the bed or do the dishes (or whatever you chose). Once the wave of fear goes over us and we realize that we survived, our brain may freak out a little less each time.

As you know, having a child is going to turn your schedule on its ear, so can you start getting used to not getting everything done perfectly and being okay with it now? One of my clients did this by not making her bed and not doing the dishes. She sat in the discomfort of it and felt into what she was making it mean: "Does it mean I will become a slob and will end up on a reality show about hoarding if I don't do these things for one day? That my life will spiral into a pit of despair? Can I prove to myself and to the Universe that I don't need to control everything?" This process really helps us to be more okay with the timing of things. Think of it as a show of commitment to do these practice runs, despite your uneasiness about them. I am of course not saying to never do dishes or laundry again; it's more about addressing the anxiety that comes up around the *need* to do it that we want to ease.

If you're reading this book, you're probably open to the idea of how your energy affects your body/life. So you may even be aware that trying to control everything is not so conducive to this process and you may want to let go of the control. We will go into the energy of this more in chapter 4, but basically most of us try to let go of our control as fast as we can—which means we are controlling how we give up control, which is still controlling. It's like trying to run away from something that you've been Velcroed to. Frustrating as that may be, there are ways around it. We're going to talk about it more in the Law of Attraction material in chapter 4, but let's find a mantra around releasing control—one that doesn't have the word "control" in it. Try some of these on for size, or create one of your own that has a positive, forward feeling, and invite in the next step, versus hunting it down:

- I invite in the next step on my journey and am excited for the abundance that's coming.

- I'm choosing to be a mom and am open to the Universe's timing of when that's best for me.

- I focus on what I'd love and let the Universe take care of the pesky details.

- I'm open to receiving my gifts from the Universe in a way that I could not or did not expect.

- I'm excited to allow flow and abundance into my life.

The cool thing about a mantra is that even if it doesn't fully resonate with you, the more you say it, the more it drops down into your body. And that's when things start to change on a cellular level. So write your chosen mantra on a bunch of sticky notes and put them everywhere— fridge, bathroom mirror, night stand, laptop, etc. Get used to saying the mantra over and over. It will help to start retraining your brain.

As Type-A-vengers, we might also want to keep an eye on our brain/ ego's need to be right and to have some tangible acknowledgment that we are doing well. As Type-A-ers, we are good little students and want to know that we are executing the task at hand correctly and performing well. Our trust for our body goes right out the window, and we rely on outside measures to tell us how well we're doing. Many of you are tak- ing your temperature every morning, feeling pressured to have sex at the exact moment you find out you're ovulating, and using ovulation sticks and waiting for the smiley-face peak fertility sign to appear. If that happy face doesn't come up, we feel that we've failed; and if it does come up, we feel like we *need* to go have sex and that this *has* to be the month we get pregnant. We will go into the energy of this in chapter 4, but suffice it to say that these things can actually exacerbate your infertility.

Constant monitoring and not trusting your body pulls in more fear, more needing, and more anxiety, which is not the cushiest place for your munchkin to bake. *Your body wants to be trusted.* It knows how to do what countless women have done before you for millennia. And I get that it's hard when you've had previous experiences that make it seem otherwise. We tend to turn these past thoughts and experiences into the belief that we need things outside of ourselves to tell us when it's okay. We will cover beliefs in chapter 2, but here's my challenge to you:

Can you commit for one month to *not*

- take your temperature,

- use ovulation sticks,

- go to the fertility specialist,

- and check your CM (cervical mucus) all the time. On the one hand this is checking in with your own body, but sometimes our Type-A brains get obsessive about it. We start checking the "all-knowing" internet for what it means, and we pull in the attached wonky energy, versus the belief that "of course I can do this."

For those of you planners who feel you're already running out of time, that thought of giving up the meticulous monitoring is going to make you gulp a little. But can you show your body energetically that you can trust it? Many of my clients who started in this place are now actually able to *feel* when they're ovulating. They feel when the cramping is different from period cramps. Just the sheer idea of trusting that their body will do what it needs to do is a *huge* leap forward.

You don't need anything outside of your body to get pregnant. Commit this month to your body. See if you can connect with it, and put out to the Universe that you know that together you can do this.

7. *You're Not Where You Want to Be in Your Career*

We covered some of this in the stressful job section, so you can go back and refer to #1 as well. But I have really been surprised by the number of my clients who also end up moving their jobs as they move their fertility. Part of this can have to do with our solar plexus chakra, which is the energetic center of drive and ambition: our power center. It's the confidence of being able to complete the things we set out to do, which can be related to work and/or fertility. If we are not feeling powerful or capable in our job, it's easy to not feel capable of anything, and that can translate into your ability to create a human. When you are feeling powerful and capable, things seem to come easy to you and there isn't a heavy "efforting" feeling, because you're not feeling powerless or at the mercy of something you can't control.

Many of you are in a job you feel obligated to be in because it's what your parents thought you should do or it's all you could find at the time. And more and more I'm finding that sometimes the reason for the baby delay is that we are really supposed to be stepping into our *purpose*—not just another higher-paying job, but our purpose. Many of us are not being what we wanted to be when we grew up. It may be partially that life got in the way, or that we were influenced by others who made us feel that the thing we wanted to be wouldn't be viable, and that we would be poor and miserable if we pursued it. Alternatively, it might be that we've never allowed ourselves to really sink into what we would love to do for a living. What would light you up if you could do it every day and get paid for it? You have a unique set of talents that you came into this world with, and we want to make sure they're being used and not squandered. If you're a CEO who's supposed to be a chef, or a dental hygienist who's supposed to be a yoga teacher, there's discord in that energy. And it can throw our whole alignment off so that we literally can't receive the things that are important to us this time around. So often we have to adjust the career area first, and then once we are in alignment, the fertility easily follows suit.

My client Eliana was a teacher. She felt obligated to stay in that career, but her dream was her side business. Crafting organic bath and beauty products made her heart *sing*. She couldn't imagine how she could let the teaching pension and the 401K go, until she saw the flexibility of working from home to be with her baby and the fact that she could build an empire on this. All of a sudden her sales started picking up, and that brought her closer to being pregnant.

EXERCISE

Write a little brain dump (freeform thought, no structure) around the idea that if money didn't matter and you could do whatever you wanted for a living, what would it be? There's no structure to this—just keep writing until you feel like you're done. It's important to write it down, as your brain processes it differently than when you just think about it. Try not to judge what comes up, and don't be the "enlightened" human being that you are. Get down-and-dirty honest and list all of the things that come up, no matter how stupid or frivolous they sound. Even if your brain/ego goes to things like "that could never happen" or "no one will pay me enough just to do that," write down everything that sounds delicious for you regarding this dream job. I jokingly say to my clients, "If you want to be a lint salesman, let's find a way to do it!" The main thing for this exercise is to feel into the excitement of letting yourself dream big and noticing how it feels to entertain that you could design a career that you'd love, versus one that you feel obligated to be in.

- What would your dream job look like?

- How would you feel?

- Who would you serve?

- How would they feel?

- What would you be helping them with?

- How many hours/days per week would you work?

- Would it be from home or in an office?

- Would you work for yourself or someone else?

- What would be exciting about it?

- How do you feel in your body when you think that this dream job could actually be enough to nourish and support you?

More and more I am seeing this list turn into people's careers or purposes. Dare to dream a little. (We'll get into why that's important in chapter 4.) It may very well be that you have a hard time identifying what your dream job title would be. That's why I want you to feel into the qualities that you'd love in a job instead of trying to fit it into the box of what your brain knows or expects. When looking at your list, it's okay if you then say, "These things aren't a job." I can relate. The work I do with my private clients is a hybrid of three different modalities. What I do didn't exist before I did it either, but now I'm helping women all over the world and am filled to the brim with purpose every day. So try not to judge what comes up, but rather feel in your bones how awesome it would be if the things you wrote down appeared on your doorstep as a job that you got to do every day and that people were paying a decent amount of money for. We must start putting out energetic feelers toward our purpose, even if we aren't sure how it's going to work out or how we're going to get there. It's important that you just acknowledge that you have a purpose other than the job you're doing, and that you then take whatever steps you can toward allowing that in.

8. Money Worries

This can be a tricky one. Money beliefs can be *deeply* embedded patterns in our psyche and can really trip us up. We learn these patterns from a very early age, without even realizing it. If we had secondhand clothes or were repeatedly told that money doesn't grow on trees, etc., it can instill in us a survival pattern of there not being enough. It can elicit a really primal fear that we're going to die at any given moment if the money stream runs out. We are going to get more into the fight-or-flight response and how it physically affects fertility later on, but know that fear—especially fear around something that dictates whether or not you have shelter or food—can be a huge block. I've been there and I totally get it, that feeling of "What if I don't have enough to pay my bills?" or "I don't see how I'm going to be able to afford that." It lasted many years for me, because not only was I not aware of the pattern, but I also didn't think there was a way out of it or that there were steps I could take to shift it.

Sometimes we get so ahead of ourselves that we never move forward because we're scared of what *might* happen. Now obviously, if you're living in a cardboard box, it might not be the best idea to bring a child into the world, but most of us are not living in that scenario. So we want to separate our thoughts from what is actually true (see chapter 2 for more), so that we are not paralyzed by fear but actually allow in more abundance—which allows our body to feel safer.

EXERCISE

Write a list of what you *do* have enough money for. Include everything you can think of, from the epic to the miniscule. Can you feel into a place of being grateful for each one of those things? When we get into manifesting in chapter 4, we will see that a big piece of getting things moving is being grateful for what we do have and *feeling* into that.

Think about what you do have that isn't necessarily monetary but is helpful in terms of making your life easier, more enjoyable, and less stressful, such as a great support system of family and friends who would help when needed. Explore these areas and then take time to feel into them.

It's important not just to make a list and intellectually acknowledge these things to be grateful for. That doesn't do much in terms of moving your energy forward. What gets things snap-crackle-popping is when you feel these things in your body. That's when things begin to change on a cellular level and you attract what you want versus what you don't.

EXERCISE

Make a goal sheet for the rest of the year. (This worksheet is included in the Conceivable Tool Kit.) Break it into three-month, six-month, and twelve-month goals. Write three goals for each time period. When setting goals, we don't want to think of them in the typical sense—the drive, the competition with the self or others, or the belief that "if I don't achieve this, I've failed." What would be *awesome* to shift in your career, or what circumstances would alleviate this concern? Each goal should feel *good* and should feel *attainable*. You don't want your brain to shut off and go, "Yeah right, that's never going to happen." So make sure it sounds exciting and a little out of your comfort zone while still plausible. The great thing is that you don't have to know how the hell it's gonna happen, but just that it would be phenomenal if it did. *Feel* into how amazing it will be when three, six, or twelve months down the road you look at these goals and they all happened!

After you fill in your sheet, post it on the fridge or your nightstand and *feel into each of the goals every day*. Each day look at them and don't try to force these goals to happen, but just imagine how lit up inside would you feel if they did. What would it *feel* like in your body if that thing just showed up?

Our perception about what money is and what it means is key. When we are stuck in these embedded patterns, it can be hard to think that money isn't the root of all evil or that you'll ever have enough. The wise Wayne Dyer said that if you change the way you look at things, the things you look at change. From an energetic perspective, if we perceive an issue as heavy, it will feel heavy. If we perceive it as light, it will feel light. The less power we give money, the less we are governed by it. Can we look at money simply as wampum—as a means of exchange—and can we get to a place of not hoping but of *trusting* that the Universe will provide what we need when we need it?

Money is necessary in today's society. There's really no getting around that unless you go off the grid. But we can reframe it as something that helps us to have the experiences in life that light us up and make us happy, versus the thing we will never achieve or that holds us back. If you're living in fear that there will never be enough, there never will be. So many of us are in survival mode when it comes to money, whether it's because we actually don't have money or we are afraid of losing it. This triggers our fight-or-flight response in a big way, because money is what we use to buy our two basic needs: food and shelter. Remember that your reproductive system isn't needed when you're running from a stressful situation. So if you are stressed about being able to provide for yourself, let alone another mouth to feed, we want to reframe that ASAP. It's our beliefs (chapter 2) that are stressful, not the actual situation, so the sooner we can see what is going right with our money situation, the sooner we can move out of the dire situation. We then go from surviving life to enjoying it—and that makes a huge difference in the quality of your life, whether there's a baby or not.

9. Do You Have a Hard Time Saying No?

This factor can be related to your job, if your boss continually asks extra things of you. It can be in terms of family (especially a tight-knit one). Is a family member ill or elderly, and a lot of responsibility falls on you? Do your drama-queen friends *need* you to be there for them all the time? Again, I'm not saying ditch your friends, your sick brother, or your grandma. I *am* saying we need to establish some boundaries.

When you are that go-to person for people and you readily do what needs to be done, people keep going to you because they know it'll get done.

It's great to know you're helping people, but this is where your little brain/ego kicks in and goes, "We are taking care of everyone but ourselves. We literally cannot handle another human," and hence the endocrine system and the reproductive system get wonky or slow/shut down because your brain is already convinced that you have no time to yourself and therefore can't possibly add a baby to the mix.

So where can we set some boundaries?

As mentioned in external factor #1 with the stressful job situation, commit to staying late only one or two days a month if it's normally five. If you don't know how well that would go over, have a conversation with your boss or the HR department. Tell them it has been recommended to you that, due to a "condition" you're going through, they'd like you to limit your overtime. You can say it without going into too many details.

If you are caring for an ailing parent or grandparent and have siblings, coordinate so that you're not the caretaker every day. If you don't, ask a family friend or spouse to help or, if means allow, hire someone to give you a break for a couple of days per week. This is *not* selfish. You are not a horrible child or grandchild if you do this. Think about what their *soul* would want for your *soul*. I promise that it's not to be stressed and tired all the time because you felt obligated. They know you love them.

Help create this space for you so you can show the Universe that you can slow down your life and make room for what you want. Make space *now*. Put that energy out there. The "I'll do it later" mentality brings more "I'll do it later" energy, which we'll get to in chapter 4, and that leads to you being stuck in an energetic loop of "later."

Additionally, some of us have friends who are living in a Greek tragedy and need our urgent help all the time amid the ninety-seven other things we have going on in our lives. One of my clients and I affectionately call these people the "facehuggers" (from the movie *Alien*). You are the person who doesn't say no, so these folks just migrate right to you. They don't know how much it taxes your energy because they're so caught up in their own drama. Do you ditch these friends? Of course not.

But you can try setting a boundary of a weekly lunch or dinner date where all the beans are spilled, and then it's just occasional texting throughout the rest of the week.

You can also tell them you've got a lot of stuff going on that you're trying to process, so if you don't get back to them right away, you still love them and will be there for them as much as you can, but there's some stuff you're working through that may inhibit that.

Let your friend know that, say, between the hours of 6:00 and 8:30 p.m., you're having dinner and catching up with your husband or partner, so if something super-important comes up, she can text you after that.

Brainstorm some things to say that would feel good to you, where you're communicating to your friend, boss, or family member that you care about them *and* that there are certain things you need as well, and you appreciate their understanding of that.

Part of the fertility puzzle is claiming the worth piece. Your needs are just as important as other people's needs. You deserve and are allowed to do whatever you need to move yourself forward. There's enough to go around for everyone. *Claim that.*

Claiming your time and space doesn't make you insensitive or a bitch or a bad friend. If you don't stand up for yourself, you can't expect anyone else to. And you can't expect the people who are sucking up your time and energy to know that they're being facehuggers if they're not made aware of it. We often don't want to stir the pot or upset people, but you can say it in a loving way by letting them know that you care about them but you also have to take care of what's best for you right now. Voicing what you need is especially important for those of you dealing with thyroid conditions, which we will explore in chapter 3.

10. Are You Eating Crap?

Here's the thing about the food piece for me: it's kind of a double-edged sword in terms of this mindset/energy work for fertility.

I try to eat clean as much as I can. I eat organic whenever possible and I feel the benefits in my body. The energy I have when I'm eating well is super-noticeable. I'm definitely an advocate of the belief that if you can fight a condition with food instead of medicine or drugs, you absolutely should. There's a lot of evidence for how you can manage hormonal imbalances with food and supplements, some of which I'm going to cover here.

My concern is that, as with many of these fertility "fixes," our brain becomes obsessed with determining the right amount of beets, kale, and folic acid we should consume. We become rigid about it, like we did with the ovulation sticks, and it actually *exacerbates* the infertility. When we obsess over making sure we eat the right amount of this or believe we shouldn't have any of that, it places our body in a stressed-out place, paranoid that the coffee we just drank means we can't get pregnant this month. It's just not a helpful place to be. We want to pull the body out of its fight-or-flight mode and help it feel safe, calm, and nourished.

The following guidelines are intended to be helpful, and I encourage you to consider consulting a holistic health coach or naturopath who has a chill vibe to further your understanding of and connection with the foods that may be beneficial.

From my experience with all of my work with clients, whether or not they got pregnant wasn't dependent on whether or not they drank a cup of coffee or didn't eat the right amount of kale. It came down to their mindset shifting. Let's face it: we've all known women who don't take care of their bodies (drinking alcohol, smoking, eating fast food, taking drugs, etc.) who get pregnant, so diet really is not the be-all and end-all. But it can help if you're approaching it from a nourishing versus militant way.

So we're going to look at five things to avoid and five foods to amp up.

Five Things to Avoid

Multiple cups of coffee per day. One cup of coffee will not kill your chances of conceiving, but caffeine in general can alter your blood sugar level and overstimulate the adrenals, which can send your hormones into a tizzy.

Soda and bottled juices. These are high in sugar and can have a negative effect on your blood sugar level and hormones.

Soy products. Unfortunately most of the soy available now is genetically modified and has been shown to affect both male and female fertility. Soy has estrogen-mimicking hormones that knock your body's hormonal balance for a loop. This especially affects men in terms of low sperm count and motility, as it mimics estrogen.

Low-fat foods, especially dairy. Not only are these foods highly processed and packed with sugar, but your body actually needs fat to grow a munchkin. A 2007 study from Harvard showed that women who ate full-fat products had a much easier time conceiving than those who consumed fat-free ones (see "Diet and Lifestyle in the Prevention of Ovulatory Disorder Infertility," www.ncbi.nlm.nih.gov/pubmed/17978119). If you feel uncomfortable about the idea of giving up low-fat foods, we need to have a look at your body image and beliefs about pregnancy. Sometimes releasing those things can be helpful so that we can physically and mentally allow a baby in.

Alcohol. Again, a glass of wine on occasion won't kill you, but if you have a glass or more every day, you might want to consider reducing or stopping altogether. Alcohol consumption can prevent the production of progesterone in women and decimate sperm count in men. Cutting out beer is what helped Chloe's husband get his count back up, and subsequently they got pregnant. So if your husband or partner drinks regularly, *at least* have him cut down when you're ovulating—but preferably stop.

Five Foods to Amp Up

Leafy greens such as spinach and kale are high in folate for healthy ovaries and vitamin E for healthy menstrual cycles.

Eggs (including the yolks) are rich in vitamin D, supporting ovulation.

Sunflower seeds are packed with zinc, which helps support egg quality. **Oysters** are also a good source of zinc.

Wild salmon has the least amount of mercury of all fish and is a great source of omega-3 fatty acids, which help to balance your reproductive system and send more blood to the necessary organs.

Nourishing herbal infusions of red clover and linden flower are helpful to both regulate hormones and reduce inflammation. (Inflammation is one of the leading causes of hormonal imbalance.) Herbal infusion recipes are included in the Conceivable Tool Kit.

Again, please don't drive yourself crazy with the exact amount of this or the wrong amount of that. If it feels good to you to do some of these things, great, but if you're spending more time and energy stressing about eating the right foods than hanging out with the hubby or taking a yoga class, then I lovingly say, "Step away." Getting too rigid about *anything* isn't good, as we mentioned before with the ovulation sticks and temperature, etc.

It's really about where your mindset and energy are. These are just supplemental suggestions.

11. Do You Not Have Closure on
One or More Relationships?

This factor might seem kind of out of left field, but a surprising number of my clients have energy hanging back in past relationships.

For some, it's the "one that got away" mentality. They wonder if they would still be together if X circumstances hadn't torn them apart, so a little stream of energy is hanging back there in "what if." This can be a tricky one to catch, because even if 95 percent of you gets that he wasn't the right guy for you, the brain can still be like, "But maybe it could have been. Maybe it would have been easier to get pregnant." As long as we've got even 5 percent of our subconscious energy in that thought, it can be enough to derail us from Operation Baby.

For others, it's not that they still want to be with the person, but that they never got closure and want to know why. *What's wrong with me that you broke up with me?* Some of my clients have subconsciously made it mean something about their worth that this person no longer wanted to be with them. Of course it's not about you or your worth, but it can feel like it, and a strand of energy is held back there. To your brain, it feels like "it shouldn't have happened this way." We'll get into why that's not so helpful in chapter 2, but trust that it actually happened the exact way it was supposed to. As long as we're sending strands of energy to "it shouldn't have happened," we keep ourselves in a sort of bizarre state of limbo. The body and the brain are inextricably linked, so if we're having these thoughts that aren't helpful, it's preventing our body from functioning at an optimal level as well.

Finally, for some others it's not that they want to be back with the person, but they are mad that they spent what they feel were their prime baby-making years with the ex. They feel that they wasted time, and now they're getting screwed because they waited too long. This is pretty common among my clients who are in their forties and had a non-committal boyfriend throughout their thirties and feel like they are being punished now that they want to have a baby with their current partner. There tends to be a lot of subconscious anger around this, which can manifest in the form of cysts, fibroids, or endometriosis (see chapter 3). It's important to address these hurts and beliefs so that your body can resume normal functioning.

You are *always* where you're supposed to be.

We have beliefs about what should have been, which we'll cover in chapter 2. But see if you can entertain letting go of the energy you're giving to him for having wasted your time. It's not affecting him. It's affecting *you*. You can't be in the energy of needing closure from him *and* be ready to make a baby at the same time. Those two energies are too far apart.

EXERCISE

Write a letter to this person. Handwrite it and get down and dirty with your emotions. Cry and yell while you're writing it. Get everything out that you need to say and then burn or shred the letter in a ceremonial "I'm done."

Visualize a gold cord of energy going from your heart to his. Sit in the emotion of this for a minute. Feel the hurt, regret, etc., and then see if you can genuinely wish him well on his path and thank him for lessons learned. (Remember, we are presented with the partners we need at the time.) Chop the cord with your hand. You may need to do this a few times to really feel a release, so rinse and repeat as necessary.

Write a brain dump (freeform thought, no structure) on why it was *purposeful* that things happened *exactly* the way they did. Why is it great that you didn't end up with him? Why was the timing not right? Why is your current partner best for you to have a baby with, and why will he be a great father? This is perhaps the most important one to feel into. Make sure you write it all down. There's something about the act of writing down your thoughts and then seeing them on paper that can help your energy shift.

Our brain loves to be in shoulda-coulda-woulda mode, but the fact is that it just keeps us stuck. We can't change the past or predict the future. The only thing we can change is the present, by choosing positive thoughts. In order to start thinking positively on a more consistent basis, we must be willing to give up our attachment to the past. This can be easier said than done, which is why doing the belief work in chapter 2 can be really helpful in terms of offloading the energy that isn't helpful to you.

12. Do You Have Space for This Baby?

A surprising number of my clients haven't given any thought to where the baby is going to go (in terms of physical space). I get it. It's one of those things where you think, "Well, we'll figure it out when we have the baby," or "I don't want to get my hopes up and then find out I can't have one." We want to get more of your energy moving toward the idea that this baby is in fact coming. We want to be able to create the physical space as well as the energetic space for the baby to come.

Many women I've spoken with are currently living in small one-bedroom apartments and haven't gotten excited about how they're going to decorate because there's nowhere for the baby to go. I get that you can't exactly justify selling your tiny apartment at the moment or converting the office right now, but if you found out you were pregnant today, where would that munchkin go?

I'm not saying to set up the crib right now. That's too much of an energetic gap for your brain to be able to get behind. *But* we want to start thinking in terms of the fact that this baby *is* coming. Doing visualizations can help you start to feel that in your body. We'll explore in chapter 4 why it's important to be putting out the energy of excitement, and that it's a matter of *when* this baby comes, not *if.*

EXERCISE

Close your eyes and take a deep breath. In the space you're currently living in, where is your baby's crib going? What about her
dresser? Changing table? Rocking chair? Really picture it. What
does it feel like to see it all set up? What do you notice in your
body when you realize that having those things set up in your
space means that *you did it*, that *she's coming*?

Is there stuff you're going to have to get rid of in order to make
room for her, things that are no longer serving you and that you
haven't used in a year or more (and probably won't)? Commit to
purging at least five things this week to symbolically make room
for the baby. See where you can commit to making even a small
change. This will go a long way in terms of shifting your energy.

My client Vicky had a tiny one-bedroom apartment, and even though
she kept it very neat and minimalist, there just wasn't enough space for
a family. Despite this, she made a plan for where she was and then began
visualizing the bigger apartment she'd love. She started a Pinterest board
and vision board without knowing how she'd convince her husband to
move. But she held the intention without attachment, and one day her
husband came home and said that he'd been looking at apartments and
was thinking they should move. Soon after they did, she was pregnant!

13. Did You Just Start a Business and
You Have to Tend to It Like a Baby?

There are so many moving parts to tend to when you're starting your
own business. Even if you are generally a laid-back person, it can be pretty
overwhelming. Even if the business is something you really love and are
passionate about, it takes a ton of energy. If we then overwhelm ourselves
with "Why can't I get pregnant?" we can be in for a serious uphill battle.

Have you found that your business *is* your baby? You provide for it, nurture it, and put its success above all else. Your brain may very well think you already have a baby and it doesn't see the need for another one. According to your brain, you're already devoted to something. From the flight-or-flight perspective, if your energy is tapped out, your brain isn't going to want to add another thing to your plate and make it harder for your survival.

So what can we do about it?

EXERCISE

We want to look at streamlining your business, whether it's how you're scheduling things or how much you take on. Can you hire an assistant or intern to take some of the menial jobs off your plate? Or can you commit to not answering anything business-related on weekends?

Implement some of the grounding techniques we talked about in the stressful job section (external factor #1), such as meditation, yoga, dancing, knitting, taking a bath, connecting to the earth, etc.

Give yourself the space to do what you need to do to feel solid in the business, and know that the baby will come when the initial craziness is over.

As women, we feel we need to do it all, and all at once. That's admirable, but not very practical. Give yourself the space and permission to have one baby at a time. You only *think* you're running out of time. I promise you're not. Building your business is great! It's going to provide a secure situation for you and your munchkin. It's okay to build it first. We'll talk about this more later on in the book, but the more in alignment you are in one area, the more the other areas are inclined to follow. Almost all of my private clients have either shifted jobs within their field or shifted fields completely, and that's when they get pregnant. By working on stepping into their purpose career-wise, it moved their fertility energy along.

When you're feeling capable and fulfilled in one area, other areas naturally begin to fall in line. Building a business, if that's what you're doing or want to do, can't be rushed. It's going to allow you amazing flexibility when you do have a baby, and you want to have as many of the kinks worked out as possible. The more you can look at it as something that's going to support you and make your life easier in the long run, the faster things will fall into place. See the act of building your business as actually helping the baby get here, because it is.

14. Do You Have a Doctor or Care Provider That You Aren't Comfortable With?

Here's the thing: I am not anti-doctor. I think many elements of Western medicine are awesome and necessary, and in a lot of cases it's good they exist. Medical science has done some truly amazing things.

My hang-up involves the seriously overlooked mindset component to physical conditions and fertility. There's a reason that IVF only works 25 to 50 percent of the time. And it's not because you had that cup of coffee you shouldn't have. It has so much to do with the mindset of the woman and what she's believing or committing to.

Thanks to the Law of Psychophysical Response, for every thought the brain has, the body has a physical or chemical reaction. So if we're having a stressful or panicked thought, it registers in the body. Thanks to the fight-or-flight response in the amygdalae of the brain, when we are stressed-out or triggered, our nonessential body systems slow or shut down. The reproductive system is not necessary for us to stay alive, so that's one of the first to be affected. Many things can trigger this response, but what I've found in my practice is that women are often plugged into beliefs that are spewed at them from society, family, and, yes, care providers. We'll get more into this in the belief and energy work later in the book, but the way some doctors, nurses, and technicians speak to women can be abhorrent and can actually perpetuate the infertility.

These are things doctors have actually said to my clients:

- Wow, you're starting late. Well, there are lots of old moms now.

- Let's just start right off with IVF. The other stuff doesn't really work anyway. (This client was completely healthy, with a regular cycle, by the way.)

- IVF probably won't even work for you, but you can try if you want.

- I doubt you have enough eggs at this point, so maybe you should look into other options.

- I mean, we *can* do an IUI right now, but it probably won't work.

- *Doctor comes in from other exam room and says:* Whew, the girl before you had eighteen follicles! But you have … three. That's good.

- You don't want to get your hopes up. You *are* over thirty.

While care providers rarely mean to be insensitive, they're often not aware that what they say and how they say it subconsciously plants itself into our belief systems—and sabotages our belief in ourselves and our body's ability to be able to do the job women have done for millennia.

The wellness aspect and bedside manner have unfortunately gone out the window in many cases. Whether that's due to training or hospital constraints, I don't know. But the focus is often on the pathology, not the person. Many just look at you as a uterus and not a human. Again, I know some warm, caring doctors, but almost all of my infertility clients have had unfortunate experiences with insensitive care providers. And because these care providers are authority figures, these women buy into the belief that they are *not* capable, that it's *not* likely to work, that they *are* too old. And according to the Law of Attraction, like energy attracts like energy, so if we're plugged into the belief that we are not capable, the Universe answers with situations that are an energetic match to that thought. The result is several rounds of IVF that don't work, unexplained infertility, etc., and it just never happens.

Of course these doctors' concerns have some basis. But unfortunately they are trained to focus on the exception, not the rule. In Europe, it's not so unusual for a woman to conceive up to age fifty. Part of that is due to eating less processed crap, and part of it is not being made to feel incapable at age thirty. Yes, it's true that your egg count goes down quite a bit after thirty, and so from a scientific perspective, the odds decrease. But that's just it—they're odds. And you need *one* egg. Just one.

When the mindset component (the idea that by shifting your thoughts, you can shift your physical condition) is left out of fertility, it can be a bleak prognosis. Your mind is so powerful. I've seen amazing things in my practice, including the following:

- Cysts and fibroids disappearing

- Scar tissue being released

- Cycle returning after years of amenorrhea

- Egg quality increasing

- Endometriosis disappearing

- Uterine lining doubling in thickness

- Thyroid conditions disappearing

- Stopping miscarriage

It all happened when the woman was open to the idea that things could be different from the prognosis they were given, by doing the work and by having a care provider who made them feel safe.

What's often overlooked throughout this fertility journey is your own intuition. You know your body better than anyone. You know what's normal for you, what feels right/wrong, etc. Unfortunately over the last few generations we've lost touch with our confidence in our intuition and have given our power over to the authorities. It's so important that you get back in touch with your intuition and start to trust it. It will help you exponentially to achieve your goal.

So many of my clients have stayed *way* too long with doctors who have made them feel uncomfortable, too old, less than, incapable, and like a lost cause. It's so subtle that you often don't notice it, but it's a *huge* factor in your progress. So if you don't *love* your doctor and they're not *uber*-supportive of your journey and what's right for you, consider a naturopath or midwife for well-woman care. If having a medical doctor makes you feel better, interview a few more and get someone you feel safe and comfortable with.

Feeling comfortable and capable is *essential* in this journey. Don't be afraid to change providers. If they're not on Team You, they need to go.

15. Are There Some Body Issues Coming Up?

This can be a big factor and may have many layers to it. After all, body image is something we're sort of forced to be aware of from a young age. If we have beliefs that are either ours, our parents', or society's that are clouding our view of ourselves, we can have a fertility block. I have several clients who are former bodybuilders, or have dealt with eating disorders, or grew up overweight and are scared to death to go back to that place.

It's not something we really want to admit to ourselves because, of course, we want the baby. This can lead to not eating well or eating processed low-fat foods, which adversely affect your hormones, as we mentioned earlier. If the hormones are off kilter or there's inflammation in the body, the chances of conceiving are significantly diminished.

We're afraid of growing larger, and that can trigger fear and kick up our Type-A desire to control how things will go, rather than basking in the idea that we're about to be pregnant. These are two conflicting energies that sort of cancel each other out.

EXERCISE

Here are some avenues you can explore to help you move through your fears around weight gain/body image.

- Consider speaking with a therapist for a couple of sessions to work through the fear.

- Check in with a holistic health coach for advice on how to eat safely and healthy as you prepare for pregnancy.

- Know that not everyone gains sixty pounds during pregnancy. In fact, twenty-five to thirty-five pounds is the typical weight gain—and if you plan to breastfeed, it comes off even quicker.

- Look into prenatal yoga classes in your area.

- Look at some of the really cute maternity wear they have now. Start to get excited about being a chic preggo mama!

- Talk to your friends who didn't take long to lose weight after giving birth and ask for their secrets.

- Come up with an accountability plan postpartum that can quell fears now, such as a walking buddy, a postpartum mommy group, a mommy and me yoga class, etc.

- Make a list of your fears and then run them through the Belief Sheet in the Conceivable Tool Kit (which we will discuss in chapter 2) to quell your anxiety.

- Make a list of the negatives of gaining twenty-five pounds and a list of the positives of having a baby. If the negatives outweigh the positives, then there might be some mindset work and healing that needs to happen before the munchkin makes an entrance. It's okay and necessary to heal this first so that you can have a beautiful, stress-free pregnancy.

Written inquiry can really help the brain release anxiety. It allows us to let go of a fear that's not moving us forward.

Body image isn't necessarily something we think of as being a factor in why we're not getting pregnant, but it's a sneaky subconscious block that can keep us in limbo. For example, my client Kelli told me in an early session that she had decided she was going to adopt. Adoption is a great option and the people who do it are heroes, but I also know that Kelli really wanted her own biological child, so I asked why. One of the first things she said was that then she wouldn't have to worry about losing the baby weight. Her friend at work who had a two-year-old still hadn't lost the weight, and she was scared that she would have the same fate. So the brain says, "Let's just adopt because it'll be easier on our body." I reminded her that she would never let the same thing happen to her. It's just not in her personality. This is where she would use her Type-A-ness for good and schedule workouts, go for stroller jogs in the morning, and cook healthy meals. She relaxed after that, which is part of what helped her get pregnant. Kelli now has a two-year-old and is actually *below* her pre-pregnancy weight!

Look over the fifteen external factors affecting fertility again, and circle the top three that you think apply to you. Take some time to write down what actions you will take to move those factors forward. You don't have to know how to "fix" the whole situation. Just put your energy forward toward what would feel really good.

2

....

Mindset Matters

How your thoughts and beliefs can get in the way of pregnancy

We're going to talk about beliefs and how they affect your fertility. We'll be breaking down what they are, why they're important, and how to start moving through them.

This is one of *the* most important pieces for moving forward at a much faster pace than with therapy or energy work alone, and it applies to all areas of your life, not just fertility. It can help with relationships, money, health... *everything*.

When I say "You might be plugging into beliefs that aren't serving you anymore," what does that mean?

What is a belief?

A belief is an acceptance that a statement is true or that something exists. Notice that I didn't say it's a truth. It's an *acceptance* that something is true. A belief is a thought you think over and over and over again until it becomes a truth for *you*. And even though it might *feel* true, I can promise you, if it's stressing you out, it's not true. Now, that's a tough pill to swallow for most people, but let me show you what I mean.

Most of my intuitive work with my private clients involves identifying these unconscious beliefs that are playing in the background. We either didn't know they were there or thought we'd already dealt with them.

Our brain's function at its very core is to keep us alive. While the fight-or-flight response still has its purpose in our lives today, it sometimes goes a little overboard. It can stop us from doing things we want or need to do because it perceives them as a threat to our "alive-ness." Whenever we start to think outside the box and want to try something that our brain has no proof we will survive, it freaks out. It sends the message that it's not safe, so we resign ourselves to not do it.

The brain begins throwing us thoughts that are way scarier than what actually *is* happening. We get so scared that we begin to think it *is* happening or that it's imminent, and we shut things down. This includes a physical shutdown, ladies. The terms *psychosomatic* and *mind over matter* exist for a reason. The mind is *uber*-powerful. I'll get more into the emotional/physical connection later in the book, but when your brain is in freak-out mode, it can slow or even stop the functioning of the endocrine system (especially the thyroid) as well as the reproductive system.

Your brain may throw thoughts at you such as these:

- Everyone says you're getting too old, so maybe you are.

- You won't have enough money to raise a child.

- You probably don't have enough eggs to be able to do this on your own.

- You should be pregnant by now.

- You're running out of time.

- Getting pregnant is hard.

- You've had a miscarriage before, so you will likely have one again.

- The world is such a dangerous place to raise a child nowadays.

These all feel defeating, overwhelming, hard, and scary. I would bet that if you've been trying to get pregnant for any length of time, more than one of these ideas has crossed your mind.

Here's where they can get you into trouble:

When we have a hard time getting pregnant, whether it's miscarriages or just a bunch of negative pregnancy tests, our brain says, "See?! It's *been* hard, so it's going to continue to *be* hard. Let's just back off." Then this thing that you want more than anything in the world slips a little further away as more of your energy says, "I guess you're right." We don't even realize what we're doing because the belief feels *so* true.

The more we plug into these thoughts and beliefs as truth, the more they begin to carve a different path for our life—different from what we want or deserve.

We are so plugged into the gripping fear that these scary thoughts will happen that we get more desperate and more attached to *needing* our thing to work out. We're going to get deeper into the Law of Attraction as it applies to fertility in chapter 4, but for now you need to know that fear and desperation attract more fear and desperation. That's all we can see. It keeps our wheels spinning in the stagnant energy of "I should be pregnant by now. When will it happen?"

As I mentioned earlier, whenever we think something *should be* or *shouldn't be* other than what it *is*, it's not true. When you're in "what is," you're okay. You're alive, and your future isn't written yet. Even if what is isn't what you want, you're coming from a more grounded, centered place to say, "Okay, this sucks right now, but it's happening. And whatever is happening is *supposed* to be happening, so let's figure out why."

I promise that if you inquire from an exploratory place of "Huh. This is weird and unexpected. I wonder what's going on," versus "Why, God, *whyyyyyy*?" you're going to find the answer a lot faster.

When you have your wheels spinning in "It shouldn't be happening like this, it should be happening like this," *so* much of your energy isn't going forward. Your body is tight and scrunched up; your emotions are raw and heightened. It's exhausting! No wonder there's not enough energy to go forward. A lot of it is committed to what you think should have happened already. Many times we aren't even aware that these thoughts and beliefs are affecting us. They're running subconsciously in the background without our awareness, like those apps on your phone, draining your battery because you haven't closed them out. When you have too much going on *and* you're constantly funneling energy to something that may or may not happen, your drained body can't do the things you want or expect it to do. Working through these beliefs and stopping the energy leak is crucial.

We can think that we "should have been pregnant by now" all day long, but the fact is, it hasn't happened yet. When your brain thinks "Pregnancy should have happened already," it makes the calculation that you've missed your window of opportunity. Since the body takes direct orders from the brain, if your brain says you've missed your window, then there's no point in your body making any effort to make this baby happen. See if you can take yourself out of your brain, look objectively at this "you" creature, and inquire what is going on that is impeding this at the moment. What steps can you take to move your energy forward? If motherhood should have happened by now, it would have. It hasn't. So why not? Explore.

Review that 15 External Factors worksheet from chapter 1. Adjustments can be made that will shift your energy forward.

Most importantly, know that there's *always* a reason for all of the challenges we face. The Universe is not random.

Without searching the internet like a maniac (which isn't good energy-wise, either), come from an exploratory place of "Ohhhhh, that's why this is happening. It's not good, it's not bad, it just *is*. And here's something I can do to move in the direction of what I want."

It's like when you have a dream that a monster is chasing you. The more you run, the more it keeps chasing you. But if you stop and turn around, you see it's not as scary as you thought and doesn't want to kill or eat you at all. It was just bringing something to your attention. We want to see the brain not as the enemy but as this scared little thing, albeit a pain in the ass, that's having a nightmare. We want to explain to it why moving forward is safe and beneficial for everyone. Then it can relax and go to bed.

It takes much less energy to come from that place and allows you to move forward *so* much quicker. It can be a little scary to entertain the idea that we can choose/are choosing everything that comes into our existence. Most people don't want that responsibility. That's where ignorance is bliss, and blaming God or the Universe takes the onus off us: "If it's God's or the Universe's fault that it's not happening, then at least it's not my fault." Or we go into a place of blaming ourselves and feeling like a worthless failure. It's no one's fault. I promise that it's actually an amazing thing that you can choose/are choosing everything that comes into your existence. Because if you are choosing, you can un-choose or choose something else that you *do* want. By shifting your beliefs, you can literally shift your reality.

The other important thing to remember is that just because it hasn't happened yet *doesn't mean it won't happen.* That's something a lot of women subconsciously believe. When you plug into that as truth, then it becomes the reality. But is it a truth on its own? No.

Here's where we have to draw a line in the sand and acknowledge that what happened in the past is *valid* and *purposeful* but that the past doesn't dictate the future unless you let it.

So how do you not let it? With a little underused thing called intuition and a worksheet.

Theoretically, if you're reading this book, you are aware of your intuition on some level. It's such a *huge* part of the work. We've heard the phrases "she's an intuitive" or "a woman's intuition," but most people have very little personal experience with intuition, let alone know how to use it to get what they want.

Intuition is defined as the ability to understand something immediately, without conscious reasoning, or as a thing one knows or considers likely from instinctive feeling rather than conscious reasoning.

I'm sure some of you have gotten a feeling or message to do, or not do, something. You couldn't explain it, but you just knew you should listen to it, and it turned out to be right. Many of us had a knowing feeling when we met our spouse—that they were the one for us. Or we've gotten an uneasy feeling that we shouldn't walk down a certain street though we couldn't explain why. Or how many times have we smacked ourselves on the head and said, "I should have listened to my intuition!"

We aren't encouraged to lead from our intuition in today's society. As women, we have been trained to default to trusting the white coats—especially around pregnancy and birth. We are told that we need to look to doctors and specialists for answers, and that our bodies aren't capable of becoming pregnant and giving birth without outside help.

Our overscheduled lives keep our brain running the show. Our poor intuition can't get a word in edgewise.

I may eventually write a whole book on intuition because there's so much to it, but here's how it applies to this belief chunk:

I like to refer to the *brain/ego* as "thinking" and the *intuition* as "knowing."

When you're trying to "think" of an answer, it's more of that forcing energy: "I have to figure it out, I have to figure it out. It shouldn't be this way! How can I get pregnant? I'll never get pregnant." That's the wheel-spinning energy.

The intuition is a knowing that you can't explain—you just know. Put a hand on your heart or your belly and take a big breath in through your nose and out through your mouth. Visualize a ball of light at the top of your head dropping into your body and slowly down to the base of your spine. It not only stops the tornado in your brain but also allows thoughts such as these: "I'm perfectly healthy. I'm still of childbearing age. I'm going to be a great mother. I get to decide the experiences I want in my life. There's no reason I can't have a baby. I know my body and myself and I know that, despite what other people may say, I can do this." It's calmer, takes less energy, and is so empowering. We have *way* more power than we use or know how to use.

I've seen amazing things happen when women are plugged into the *knowing* versus the *thinking* place. All of my clients who got pregnant succeeded through getting to that *knowing* place.

Your brain is super-adept at keeping you out of harm's way, and although it means well, it can be really sneaky. So it's going to take a while for *you* to get more adept at using your intuition to counter and move through the brain's freak-outs.

While you're getting more adept at that, we can use the Belief Sheet from the Conceivable Tool Kit to delve into the brain's fears and the intuition's empowerment.

This Belief Sheet is adapted from "The Work" by Byron Katie. She developed an amazing inquiry of our stressful thoughts that can stop years of anguish in minutes, available for free at her website, TheWork.com. When I began using it, I couldn't believe how it helped my relationship, finances, and future interactions that might otherwise have derailed me. It can move you forward much faster when you really allow yourself to "go there."

When filling out the worksheet, you don't want to be the enlightened human being that you are. You want to get down and dirty with fear, pettiness, anxiety, and anger. And *feel* it, don't *think* it.

When starting this work, some people are scared that if they really go there with the emotion, they'll attract more if it. And this piece is different from the Law of Attraction in the sense that we need to feel it in order to be able to let it go. Too often we've been shoving these feelings down. From an energetic perspective, which we will get to in chapter 4, if you're pushing these feelings down, that means they're coming up—which means you're pushing them down, which means they're coming up. It's exhausting for your mind and body to do this for any length of time. It's time for these feelings to surface and be processed so they can let go of us. Then it becomes something that happened *for* us and not *to* us.

The turnaround at the end of the Belief Sheet brings the positive that we're looking for, so please go full bore with this part. Otherwise it's like putting a bandage on gangrene. We need to dig out these uncomfortable emotions and beliefs and deal with them. (We will discuss the turnaround portion of the Belief Sheet in more detail shortly.)

The brain and its beliefs can be sneaky. They are that elevator music you don't even realize is playing in the background. Your brain is perfectly happy that you're not aware they're only thoughts. To you they seem real, and therefore you aren't able to move forward. And with that, the brain has won, because that way you're safe and alive, so the brain has done its job.

When working with my private clients, I'm able to tap into the specific beliefs that are holding them back. Here is a list of the **nine most common beliefs I see coming up for women struggling with fertility:**

- I'm running out of time/I'm too old.
- I wasted my prime baby-making years.
- I'm going to get my period…again.
- Getting pregnant is hard.
- I should be pregnant by now.
- I'm being punished for a previous termination(s).
- I'm never going to get pregnant on my own.
- I've miscarried before, so I will again.
- If I'm positive about it, I'll be more disappointed when it doesn't happen.
- I have _____ condition, so that means I can't have a baby on my own.

We aren't preprogrammed with these beliefs; *they are learned.* We "download" them from our previous experiences, including those with our parents, teachers, peers, doctors … the list goes on. Sometimes it's hard to tell where they came from because they're so ingrained. Many are society's beliefs, so we end up living in this weird "brain cult" where everyone accepts the fears as true when they're really not.

It can seem hard or nearly impossible to extract yourself from the scary thoughts, but by doing this worksheet you can take the personal, scared element out of the thought and really look at it from a place of objective inquiry. While a belief sheet can be done at any time, I suggest not doing one when you're amped up about a belief. It may still help, but chances are your brain will be so freaked out that it will try to rationalize and convince you that it has worked it out and everything's all better when it's not. You're more likely to "think" the answer than "feel" it. That's really the tricky part.

It may seem like walking a fine line, but if you truly go there and dig, the same problem cannot show up in the same way again. There may be several legs to a certain belief that sound similar, but that particular belief, if fully worked and felt through, will let go of you for good. The best time to go through these beliefs is when you're not supercharged about them.

This is where a lot of people get confused and say, "Well, I don't think this way all the time, so do I really need to work on the belief?" The answer is *hell to the yes.* The brain is awesome at convincing you that you've got it under control and it's not that big of a deal. It's perfectly happy for you to not deal with your issues, so it goes on playing in the background without you noticing until (cue ominous, scary music!) it's the fourth week of your cycle and you are a scared, desperate maniac. It's hard to back down from that attachment and truly plug into your intuition when you're not used to doing so. It's a work in progress, but know that when you "need" something to happen, that's the best way for it not to happen.

Just a side note about referring to it as "the week of your period": This is an energetic thing that we'll get into in chapter 4, but if you're referring to it as "the week of your period," the Universe is hearing that you're expecting your period to come. See if you can start looking at it as "test week."

When you're doing the Belief Sheet, look at the question "How do you feel when you think that thought?" We know you're not thinking it *all* the time. Tune in to the times when you *are* thinking that thought. Use your cell memory and your imagination. When you're in that thought spiral, what is going on?

Similarly, when you get to "Who/How would you be if you COULDN'T think that thought? How would you FEEL in your body and show up in life?" use your imagination. If nothing was actually wrong, how would you feel? Your brain's default answer is going to be "I don't know," so press further. If you *did* know, how would you feel?

Imagination and creation are technically different but are tightly linked, and the more you can go there with your imagination, the easier it is to access and begin trusting your intuition. Creativity and children are both represented by the sacral chakra. The more open to creativity and imagination you are, the wider the doorway for your munchkin to come in.

When beginning this work, most people have a hard time with the turnaround portion of the belief sheet. We want to look for three statements where the *opposite* of the belief could be true and three examples of where each of those turnaround statements could be true. The idea is that if you're finding multiple examples of where the opposite of your belief is true, then your belief can't be true.

Here is an example of the belief work I did with one of my clients, using a belief sheet. Sometimes these can be difficult to do on your own. I will often dig a little deeper when working with clients, but the Belief Sheet is a great tool to use on your own or with a mentor who will hold you accountable. I wanted to include this to illustrate how the process works with a real-life situation.

Maria's belief statement: *I'm probably going to get my period this month.*

Is it true? Yes.

Can you be 1,000 percent sure that you're probably going to get your period this month (feel into it)? No.

How do you feel when you think that thought? (Close your eyes and notice your muscles, breathing, where that feeling shows up in your body): I feel it in my lower abdomen. Nervous butterflies. Panic. Fear. Resigned. Really sad. Defeated. Dread.

How do you show up in your life when you think that thought? What/How does it affect your life when you think that thought? I'm scared and on alert all the time. I alternate between that and the feeling of "What's the point of trying?" I'm not present. I'm in the future with something I'm convinced will happen, but I really don't know if it will or not. I've got a bit of a wall up—not wanting people to ask me how it's going or feeling sorry for me because I can't seem to manage this one simple task. So I withdraw from other people, from my husband, from the whole process.

Who/How would you be if you COULDN'T think that thought? How would you FEEL in your body and show up in life? Lighter. Like I can breathe a little easier. Excited butterflies in my stomach. If I couldn't think that I was probably going to get my period, I'd be excited that this could be the month. I'd be looking forward to testing, knowing that I've been taking care of myself and there's no reason I *wouldn't* be pregnant! I'd feel more confident, more present. More capable.

Which way is going to get you what you want: thinking the thought that you're probably going to get your period or not thinking the thought? Why? Not thinking the thought. Because if I have that wall up or am resigned, then I'm never going to attract what I want—only what I don't want. If I'm able to feel confident and capable, then theoretically that has an effect on my body as well. I have to at least give myself that chance. I've also projected a future that hasn't happened yet, and am kind of shooting myself in the foot before I really get started.

The turnaround. Can you find three examples of where the opposite of your belief is true? (Ex. If the belief is "My boyfriend makes me mad," these are the turnarounds: I make my boyfriend mad. My boyfriend makes *me* happy. I make me mad.): I'm probably NOT going to get my period this month. I'm probably going to be pregnant this month. It's okay if I do get my period this month.

Can you find three examples where each turnaround is/could be true?

I'm probably NOT going to get my period this month. It could be true because:

- We had sex this month!

- My hormones are normal, so there's no reason why it couldn't happen.

- The past doesn't equal the future. Just because I have gotten my period in the past doesn't mean that will always be the case. I've been taking care of myself, so I have no reason to think anything would go wrong.

I'm probably going to be pregnant this month. It could be true because:

- Similar to the first turnaround, I am taking care of myself and doing everything right, so there really is no reason to think my body will fail me this month if I just look at it as this isolated incident and not at everything that's happened in the past. I was also in a different emotional place then.

- In terms of the Law of Attraction, if I'm confident and excited and not feeling desperate, then I'm not aligned with the disappointment. My health is in order and I know I'm meant to be a mother, so why not this month? It's as good a time as any!

- I know that a lot of symptoms of PMS are symptoms of early pregnancy as well, so if I don't go there with "Oh great, here come the cramps or spotting," it could be that I'm having implantation bleeding. If I can get myself aligned with "It's all good, I can do this, all these signs are good," then it's entirely possible I could be pregnant.

Sometimes there will be a turnaround that makes you go "*Huh*? That sounds awful!" For example, take a look at the last turnaround: "It's okay if I do get my period this month." Your initial reaction might be "It's *not* okay!" But how, theoretically, *could* it be okay? The purpose of this is not to set you up to fail; it's to help you let go of the attachment energy that you *have* to be pregnant this month—because that brings more attachment, as we will see in chapter 4. We want to be as neutral as possible, because everything that happens is happening for us—even when it's not the timing we think it should be. So how *could* it be okay?

It's okay if I do get my period this month. It could be true because:

- Maybe we have a really busy couple of months coming up at work and it would be hard for me to be newly pregnant right now. If it's not happening this month, it's not supposed to.

- There's something else I'm supposed to be working on first, so I'll explore that and trust that it'll happen when it's supposed to.

- It gives me an opportunity to work through some of these beliefs and learn more about how I'm putting my energy out there. It gives me time to let go of this attachment and amplify my intuition, which will help me in every area.

- If I do get my period, it *is* going to be okay. No one is going to die. It's not a "this month or nothing" scenario, despite my brain's efforts to make it appear that way. I do technically have time beyond this month.

This gives you an idea of how the process works. Look at your list of beliefs or sit with your intuition, and see what beliefs are coming up for you. Then run them through the Belief Sheet. The important thing is to take your time with it and actually feel into the bad and the good. Remember, *feeling* helps things begin to shift on a cellular level. If you just skim it, the belief will continue to lurk beneath the surface. So you owe it to yourself to really go there. It's better to be uncomfortable for a few minutes than to suffer through years of frustration.

Learn to sit in what feels good too, because emitting that can bring more feeling good. Feeling like you need to check for spotting or temperature or peak ovulation keeps you a slave to this condition. It can seem hard to break out of that pattern, but it's absolutely possible. This belief work is a good way to do that.

Remember that if a thought is stressing you out, you're believing something about the situation that's not true. I totally get why some of these beliefs will feel so true, but see if you can step back and find how they're actually not. Taking the fear and urgency out of the situation allows you to look at the situation clearly and realize that it's only a thought. See if you can get here: "It's not actually happening to me right now. I'm safe. It's only a thought, and thoughts can be changed." That's the first step toward changing your reality.

So many of us live in the past or the projected future. The past has already happened, and we can't change it. The future hasn't happened yet, but we waste so much time in the fear of what might be when we can't possibly know if it will be true. We spend so much energy in the trauma of the past and fear of the future, but the only place we can actually change anything is in the present. When we are in "what is," we are okay. Right now we are alive, we ate today, we have a place to live—for this moment we are okay. If we let go of the "story" of what is scary or why we can't do something, we can then actually be open to solutions that can move our situation forward.

3
....

The Body as a Map

Learning to listen to the messages your body is giving you

In this chapter we'll be covering the correlation between our emotions and physical conditions in the body—specifically, of course, in terms of fertility. We will be looking at the top ten physical conditions and their emotional causes to give you an idea of what messages your body has for you. Since unexplained infertility falls under this umbrella as well, even if you don't have a physical condition or dis-ease per se, this info will still apply to you.

I'm going to present a different concept that I don't expect you to believe right away but would like you to be willing to entertain. In my research throughout the years, I've found that various cultures and teachers, from Traditional Chinese Medicine and Ayurvedic medicine to Edgar Cayce, Louise Hay, and Drs. Lissa Rankin and Bruce Lipton, talk about the correlation between your emotional system and where it shows up or manifests in your body. You can heal your body by changing your thoughts and dealing with the issue that is causing discomfort in your body.

When you have a condition that you've been told will never go away or is so painful each month that it makes you cry, it can be hard to think that by shifting your energy you can actually shift that physical condition. It can trigger some feelings of fear or anger for your brain, because it's a little scary for your brain to believe that you could actually move forward from this. So if you get triggered, see if you can find what unhealed part of yourself that's bringing up for you, because it's an opportunity to heal it. You can decide not to act, but just know that the pattern will repeat itself. So see it as a great opportunity to move out of stagnancy and pain, and entertain that things could be different. Every condition mentioned in this chapter can and has been worked through by others, so it's important to remember that you are just as deserving and capable as these women who've done it.

We can use the body as an indicator of what's going on so we can deal with this issue on a core level and get where we want to go. We tend to go to war with our body when it's not doing what we want. We become our body's fair-weather friend when we don't get the desired result. We feel as though we know best and get really pissed off when our body doesn't follow suit. Why won't it get on board? We feel that it's betraying us. But really, it's an elaborate, genius map or system trying to get our attention. Your body is brilliant and loving and just wants to show you that "Hey, there's some stuff we need to work on. I'm going to keep on you until you work through it because it's important for your growth." It's like that check engine light in the car we mentioned earlier. The problem is usually nothing terrible, but we should investigate/replace whatever is faulty if we expect the car to get us where we want to go.

The main points I want you to come away with are that your body is on your side, stop ignoring what it's feeling, and get better at paying attention so you can figure out what it's trying to tell you

We want to look at what our body is telling us as a gift rather than a pain in the ass ... or knees or whatever. How could your body actually be trying to move you forward instead of holding you back? There's always a reason. Can you come from an exploratory place to inquire and move forward rather than spinning your wheels and wishing it weren't happening?

Certain areas of the body correspond to certain emotional issues. We see varying accounts of this in acupuncture, reflexology, and so on. Perhaps the most comprehensive guides that explain the correlations between the emotional cause and the physical issue are *Metaphysical Anatomy* by Evette Rose and the glossary in *You Can Heal Your Life* by Louise Hay. The concept of there being an emotional cause for a physical issue is a key component of my work. It's a great jumping-off point to find where my clients are stuck so I can hone in further.

For example, the knees have to do with your flexibility as a person. If the feet represent the path you're on, the knees are the means by which you get there. The inability to bend and be flexible on your path will make it harder to reach your goal or destination. One of my friends blew out his ACL on a ski slope, and while, yes, the physical cause was the icy mountain, the injury was a signal of his inflexibility as a person. It was his way or the highway and his timeline, so the Universe said, "Okay, you're literally on a slippery slope and you need to learn to be more flexible"— which he is nowadays, thanks to that incident.

Another common example is the back. You may know the saying "Get a backbone." The back is your strength and supports your whole structure. The lower back is usually connected to financial fears or not feeling supported by money. This doesn't always mean that you're broke; it's more about the fear of losing money or not having enough.

We're going to hone in on fertility and the problem areas I see most in my clients, but I wanted to give you a broader idea first since most of us know someone with knee or back pain.

Open your heart and see if you can make peace with your body. If things have gone haywire, it's because something needs to be addressed. *You're not broken or cursed. It's not your fault or your body's fault. It's a gift.* Your job is to hear, interpret, and act. This moves you forward much faster than being mad or fighting with your body or wishing it were other than it is. You will only keep your brain/ego happy by spending your energy fighting instead of moving forward.

Your body is ultimately what is going to be carrying this baby, so the sooner you reconcile with it and play for the same team, the sooner the munchkin can arrive. Try to come from a curious place rather than a frustrated, "hunting down the problem" place. We'll get into why that's important in chapter 4.

EXERCISE

Pick something that's been bugging you physically. It doesn't have to be something major, like PCOS (polycystic ovary syndrome) or your thyroid. It can be a headache or the toe you stubbed earlier today. Or, if you are in the unexplained fertility group, pick that and inquire where in your body that's sitting and why.

Close your eyes and breathe slowly in through your nose and out through your mouth. See what thoughts or images bubble up without judging them. Ask your body: What is your message for me?

Be curious. You can't get it wrong. Breathe into it and ask again. Take a second and write down your initial thoughts.

If you didn't get anything, that's okay! Doing this daily will help build that muscle, and you'll be able to tune in to your body's messages and move through the issues more quickly. The main thing is that you allow an answer to come in versus hunting down the most brilliant answer ever. Let it come to you. This is part of releasing control that we talked about earlier. Allow yourself to be supported by the Universe.

Let's look at the ten most common physical issues in fertility, their emotional cause, and what you can do about them.

1. Hypothalamus and/or Pituitary Gland

Chances are, if you're having hormonal issues, the hypothalamus and/or pituitary gland plays a part in it. The main function of the hypothalamus is to link the nervous system to the endocrine system via the pituitary gland. It is responsible for homeostasis (keeping the body regulated), body temperature, hunger, fullness, circadian rhythms, balance, and release of hormones.

The pituitary gland has many functions, but the front part of it is responsible for regulating the thyroid and adrenal glands as well as the ovaries. If there's a problem with the connection here, some women won't be able to cycle on their own or will have a hard time stimulating follicles.

What's the Emotional Cause?

The hypothalamus and pituitary gland represent the control center of the brain. Sometimes the issue shows up as a result of an eating disorder, or as the result of a traumatic experience like abuse or surviving a natural disaster. If we are taught or we learn through our various experiences that we need to control things to be safe and take it to the nth degree, there may be an issue here. There is an extreme fear here of not being in control, and a need to clutch in order to control the only thing you can—your own body.

One of my clients was a bodybuilder. Traumatic past relationship experiences led to an eating disorder, which was perpetuated in her bodybuilding career. She felt out of control when her relationship ended, so she began to hypercontrol her body and what it was ingesting. When she began competing, she was hypercontrolling both the inside and the outside of her body, and her hypothalamus short-circuited, for lack of a better term. This resulted in her not getting her period for over seven years, until we started working together.

What Can You Do About It?

I'd recommend doing a brain dump and trying to find the point in your life where this need for control started. Did your parents get divorced? Did your boyfriend break up with you? Were you in a traumatic car accident?

Find how those situations where you thought you needed control were perfect and purposeful, and why you no longer "need" to hang on to the control. Actually write it out.

Then burn or shred the list as a symbolic letting go.

I also find Clary Sage essential oil by Young Living really effective in regulating the hypothalamus. Use it on the base of the brain stem (where the head meets the neck).

2. Thyroid

The thyroid regulates your metabolism, body temperature, endocrine system, and, most importantly in our case, the reproductive system. Problems here usually manifest in the form of hypothyroidism or Hashimoto's disease. Many women don't even know they have this and aren't diagnosed until they're tested. And even blood tests can be misleading, showing a normal thyroid level when it's not. If the thyroid is malfunctioning, the likelihood for conception issues increases.

Major symptoms include extreme fatigue, muscle weakness, depression, and increased sensitivity to heat or cold.

What's the Emotional Cause?

The thyroid resides at the throat chakra, which energetically concerns being able to voice your opinions and feeling that you're being heard. When you have a thyroid issue, there's likely something lacking in that department. If you're not able to be yourself or fully assert your worth, there may be an issue here.

In addition, when we're used to being good at things but we're not good at getting pregnant, there's some shame and a feeling that it's not fair around that. The emotional issue manifests in the place where you'd voice it: the throat.

Sometimes it's not just trying to get pregnant that sets off the thyroid. Some of my clients had abusive parents who humiliated them, and some are not where they want to be in their career and wonder when someone will see and value them.

What Can You Do About It?

If you're looking for a nonmedical alternative, EndoFlex essential oil by Young Living is amazing. Put it on your back, across the bottom of your rib cage, and on your throat.

Try a red clover infusion (not tea or capsules) with a pinch of mint. This regulates the hormones and can help heal the thyroid. (Herbal infusion recipes are included in the Conceivable Tool Kit.)

Do a brain dump on when this emotional cause started for you. When did you notice these symptoms? What was going on in your life at the time? What has been hard to voice, or where do you feel not seen? What's going on now that's mirroring that feeling? Feel into all of these things and see if you can choose to let them go. You can write each one on a piece of paper, feel the emotion of it, decide that it's no longer serving you, and then burn the paper.

Make a list of victories—things you have gotten to do, are good at, and have done well—so you begin to feel that getting pregnant is no different than those achievements. Place the list where you'll see it every day, and focus on what you are good at so you can bring in more of that same energy. Take each victory on your list individually, close your eyes with your hand over your throat, and say each one three times.

Have a mantra—a simple sentence that you say over and over when you're meditating, brushing your teeth, driving in your car, etc. The more you say it, the more it drops into your body and can be a great starter to realigning your thoughts. So try something like this: "It's my turn now to be pregnant. I deserve it. I choose it." Pick something that resonates with you and "speaks up" for what you'd love to happen.

My client Gemma developed a thyroid issue after two miscarriages. She was used to being good at everything, but now she felt she wasn't good at getting pregnant. We worked together voicing and processing why everything was happening for a reason. Soon after, she was pregnant and the thyroid condition was nowhere to be found. It didn't need to be present anymore because she had worked through the problem and understood why it was coming up in the first place.

3. Amenorrhea

This literally means the absence of blood, or not having a cycle. This condition can sometimes go hand in hand with the hypothalamus/pituitary gland situation we mentioned earlier.

What's the Emotional Cause?

Several of my clients with this condition were female bodybuilders and/or had an eating disorder, or had survived a traumatic event like abuse or a natural disaster.

We talked about the fight-or-flight response that happens in your body when your brain is freaked out. This involuntary reaction happens when the brain perceives a threat to the body and prepares it to fight the threat or run from it. The heart, brain, lungs, and feet are required for this. The reproductive system is not. When you're being chased by wolves, the last thing you need is to be menstruating or getting pregnant. It's not in the interest of keeping you alive for those things to be happening at such a crucial time. We're not chased by wild animals so much anymore, but our brain perceives threats just as intensely as if we were. It's a survival instinct. When we feel utterly out of control in our life and are grasping at ways to control it, that is scary enough to your brain to cease functioning of the lady parts. And it will not turn back on again until it feels safe to do so.

When it's an eating disorder, the mind-body cause is more the need to control things. Your life feels out of control, so what can you control? Everything that happens with your own body. Otherwise it tends to be more an issue of denying your feminine side. In the case of the female bodybuilders and extremely competitive women in general, they are in a masculine career and are forcing their body to extremes in weight and discipline, which is not conducive to carrying a child.

Some women with this condition have had some past trauma or abuse and it doesn't feel "safe" to them to be feminine, so their body listens and retracts its feminine function.

Others have survived natural disasters—the ultimate in being out of control. My client Valentina survived a hurricane when she was eight years old. She lost everything and barely survived the ordeal. She understandably developed anxiety and OCD over the years, which was her brain's attempt to have control over *something* when she experienced control of *nothing*. When she went into puberty, she never got her period—ever. Her body was still in enough shock from her experience at eight years old that her body deemed it not safe enough to menstruate. As we know, you need to be having a cycle to get pregnant, so this is what we worked on first. Two days after our first session, Valentina got her period. The things we talked about made her body feel safe enough to release and relax. There would still be more processing to do, but her brain feeling safe and supported allowed her body to resume normal functioning.

What Can You Do About It?

Clary Sage essential oil by Young Living is great for this condition. Several of my clients who hadn't had a cycle on their own in years or ever got one just days later after using it. Apply it to your lower abdomen and at the back of your head (where it meets the neck).

Red clover and red raspberry leaf infusions can also help regulate your hormones and your cycle. There are no contraindications. (See the recipes in the Conceivable Tool Kit.)

Saying a mantra like "It's safe for me to be a woman," "I embrace my femininity," "I'm safe," "All is well," or "I allow my healing" over and over can be helpful. Find something that resonates with you and put it on sticky notes everywhere so you'll remember to say it constantly.

See if you can find the place in your past where the amenorrhea started and determine why it wasn't safe or helpful for you to be feminine. What was going on in your life that caused you to feel unsafe or that triggered the fight-or-flight response without you realizing it? Write down all your thoughts around that time. Seeing it on paper can help your brain realize that it was an isolated incident and not a recurring threat. Thanks to the Law of Psychophysical Response, whether you're going through a trauma or reliving the thought of it, it's all the same to your brain. There's a physical reaction for every thought. See if you can zoom out of your body and figure out why it was purposeful that it happened in the grand scheme of things. Can you decide to release those things either by writing down and burning them or by having some energy work such as reiki or acupuncture to help purge it?

Make a list of what makes you feel safe and why you're actually okay, and feel into that list every day.

4. Low Egg Count/Poor Egg Quality

There's a general freak-out that as we get older, the quality of our eggs declines and therefore there can be complications with the fetus. What is not taken into consideration is the health and mindset of each individual woman, which greatly affects the quality of her eggs. There's also the freak-out that we lose 90 percent of our eggs by the time we're thirty.

But we're born with one to two million eggs. So you've still got 100,000 left, at least. And remember, you only need *one.*

What's the Emotional Cause?

This physical condition is one that is more heavily influenced by the beliefs of doctors and is generally accepted by society as being true— that we're running out of time. We better hurry up or there'll be no good eggs left! This one makes me crazy. We touched on it in chapter 1.

Ovaries represent the point of creation. When we are plugged into the belief that we're running out of time, our count can in fact drop (like sand through an hourglass). When we lose confidence in our ability to create, our ways of creating literally diminish. Why are women in European countries giving birth to healthy babies much later in life? Partly because they don't eat the same amount of processed shit that we do, and partly because they don't have the same pressure from doctors that we do.

What Can You Do About It?

Don't give in to the fear. Yes, there are some cases where there have been unhealthy births, but the fact is that *it's not the norm* and there are other factors involved besides age.

Do a belief sheet on *I'm running out of time.* We want to work this through so that we realize it's not true and we can let go of that energy and allow the body to do what we know it can—and what women in other countries are doing naturally into their early fifties.

Make a list of why you are capable of doing this—physically, mentally, spiritually.

Often when our egg count goes down, we are losing faith in our ability to create. So activating the sacral chakra, which is the creativity/children/relationship chakra, is helpful. Simply place a hand on your lower abdomen and close your eyes while visualizing a small orange ball of light spinning in this chakra.

Slowly visualize it getting bigger and brighter and spinning faster until it has filled up your entire trunk.

You can also visualize whatever you think your eggs look like in there: glowing white or gold and multiplying—puffing up like popcorn. Don't force it; just feel into the excitement that you're able to shift this physical issue by shifting your thoughts.

5. Ovarian Cysts and Fibroids

Ovarian cysts are fluid-filled sacs that sit on the ovaries. Most of the time they're harmless, but when they rupture it can be more serious. Symptoms include pelvic pain (before a period or during sex), fullness or heaviness in the abdomen, and a dull ache radiating into the lower back and thighs.

Fibroids are firm, rubbery masses on the uterine tissue. While almost never cancerous, they can wreak havoc with heavy, painful periods, prolonged periods, pelvic pressure, and constipation.

Both can affect the reproductive process.

What's the Emotional Cause?

The ovaries and uterus represent the point of creation. This is literally where life is created. It's also the location of the sacral chakra (see chapter 5 for more info), which represents relationships, creativity, and children. The mental/emotional cause for cysts and fibroids is hanging on to hurt or resentment about a situation. This usually involves wounds from past relationships, perhaps not getting closure or feeling like you wasted your prime baby-making years with that person. It can also be from a current relationship, if there's been infidelity or a big issue that hasn't really been dealt with. The relationship is most often romantic but can also include friendships, work partnerships, family, etc. Cysts and fibroids are both physically and energetically painful growths on your point of creation, and therefore they literally inhibit your ability to create (in this case, a child).

What Can You Do About It?

Trace back to when you got the cysts/fibroids (approximate if you don't know for sure). Look at what was going on in your life at the time—relationships, breakups, difficult work relationships, anger at partner or self for "wasting time," guilt (strict parents/ religious beliefs around sexuality), etc. Look at all areas of your life at that time and do a brain dump on a piece of paper. Look through each sentence and ask if it's serving you to continue to hold this in your body. Ask yourself why this challenging experience was purposeful. (It was—so see if you can figure out why, in the grand scheme of your life, it makes sense that it happened and what you learned from it.) Then either outside or safely in your kitchen sink, *burn it.* Burning the paper represents a ceremonial "I'm done and I'm choosing to move forward."

Close your eyes and visualize a white or gold cord from your heart to the other person's. Tell them how hurt you were. Say what you need to say—cry, yell, plead, etc. Then take a deep breath and see if you a can find a place where you can thank them for the lessons you learned from them and their part in your life. Let them know that you're done and moving on, and you wish them well on their path. Cut the cord by making a chopping motion with your hand. (You may have to do this several times to really connect to the feeling of it.) Put a hand over your heart and fill the hole where the cord was with warm white light and then seal it off— sort of an energetic cauterizing so that the cord from that person can't ever plug into or drain you again.

You can also try visualizing one cyst or fibroid at a time, and surrounding it with light. As you visualize it shrinking, say: "That relationship was purposeful. I release it with love and move forward." Say this several times. Visualization is such a helpful tool if you can make it work for you. One of my clients got rid of ovarian cysts this way, another got rid of scar tissue from a previous procedure in her subsequent cycle, one increased her egg quality, and one doubled her dangerously thin uterine lining—all by using visualization. Sometimes playing soothing music and/or burning sage, incense, or a scented candle can help you keep your focus.

We often are not nourishing ourselves on this journey. We are in push or survival mode more often than not. So see if you can come up with five ways to nourish yourself. They don't have to be epic, expensive things, but just little things you can do that are just for you. As one of these things, I'd suggest a linden flower infusion to reduce inflammation alternated with a red clover infusion to help regulate your hormones with zero side effects. (See the Conceivable Tool Kit for the recipes.)

My client Margot didn't realize that she was still hanging on to hurt and resentment toward the boyfriend she'd had before her husband. He had been noncommittal and had cheated on her, and she was angry that she had wasted so much time on him. We worked on processing and releasing those feelings, and her cysts and fibroids were nowhere to be found at her next appointment.

6. Miscarriage or Terminations

Many women understandably have a really hard time with miscarriages, mostly because of the loss of something they really wanted; but also it's still a hush-hush thing, and many women don't realize how common it actually is. A surprising 10 to 20 percent of first pregnancies end in miscarriage, but most of us wouldn't know that because it's kept under wraps societally, and also because we can feel like a failure and don't want people to know about our "shortcomings." This unfortunately makes our grief and healing more difficult.

The same can be said of terminations. Most people do not reach out for support or even vent their feelings, which can lead to the following emotional manifestations.

What's the Emotional Cause?

When we have had one miscarriage, it's so hard not to be freaked out about the next pregnancy making it. It's really easy to plug into the belief that because it happened once, it'll happen again. We don't know how to address the reason for the first one and are scared about having another one, so often the pattern of multiple miscarriages perpetuates. One of my clients had two miscarriages and then couldn't get pregnant again. Her brain was deathly afraid of her body being in danger a third time, so it just shut down her reproductive and endocrine systems. When miscarriages happen, the mind-body cause is fear of the future and inappropriate timing. Initially you'll think, "No, I was totally ready," but I guarantee there was a reason, if you really investigate. The same applies to terminations. Not one of my clients took that decision lightly, but most never discussed it with anyone, leaving those feelings to fester in the body and leading to the physical problem of having difficulty getting pregnant now, whether it be due to guilt or fear of karma or punishment.

What Can You Do About It?

Inquire about the following:

- Were you in a financially scary place when you had the miscarriage or termination?
- Was your relationship not stable?
- Were you in flux with your career or starting a new job?
- Did you move?
- Were you taking care of an ailing loved one?

- Are you scared to death of the birth process?

- Do you or did you have high anxiety?

Really do some searching of what your circumstances were. This will apply to both miscarriages and terminations (and the subconscious guilt we can still carry).

Write down the circumstances so your brain can really see why it didn't happen. If there were multiple miscarriages, look at each one separately. Then look at your circumstances now. Theoretically there have been some changes and you're in a better place now, and you can feel like it won't repeat itself.

If it still feels scary, pull out a belief sheet and look at *I miscarried before, so I will again*, or, for a termination, *I'm being punished for the termination by not getting pregnant now.* They're both not true, but I get why they feel true, so really *feel* into them. Don't think the answers. Feeling is how you shift.

Why Is It Perfect?

So often in this process, if we think we should have been pregnant by now or if we've had a miscarriage, we can feel that this situation isn't fair. We can feel that the Universe is against us and that it may never happen. Whenever we think something should be different from what it is, it's not true.

That's a tough pill to swallow for a lot of people, but it's all kinds of true. If it should have happened, it would have. If it shouldn't have happened, it wouldn't have. We get a little rigid about what we think is a good timeline for our stuff to materialize, but our path is so much bigger than what we are consciously aware of. So we want to look at the situation from a curious, exploratory place and say, "Okay, here's what is: I feel like I shouldn't have had a miscarriage. But if I shouldn't have, I wouldn't have. I did. So what might be going on in my life or in my experience that would precipitate that?"

For example, perhaps you moved, you got a new job, your job was stressful, your husband was out of work, your relationship was rocky, you were overscheduled at work or in your life, etc. I guarantee you there's something. Sometimes it takes looking at it on paper for your brain to go, "Ohhhhh, it couldn't have happened before now. We had X, Y, and Z going on." It's important that you release the energy you have spinning in what should have been and direct it toward what you'd actually love. Then look at why now *is* the right time for you to get pregnant. You can use these two worksheets from the Conceivable Tool Kit: Why Wasn't It The Right Time Before Now? and Why Is It the Right Time Now?

After some belief work and energy work and some coaching to work through why things had happened, my client was able to let go of the fear and get pregnant.

I find Valor essential oil by Young Living really helpful for fertility in general, but especially for alleviating miscarriage fear. Apply it to the base of your spine and the bottoms of your feet. I also recommend SARA and Release essential oils by Young Living. They're great for processing past trauma and can help with releasing the stored trauma of miscarriage or termination. A Guide to the Best Essential Oils for Fertility is included in the Conceivable Tool Kit.

7. Endometriosis

With this condition, tissue that normally grows on the inside of your uterus grows on the outside and adheres to other organs, such as the ovaries. The endometrial tissue becomes trapped, surrounds these organs, and can't be released with the normal menstrual cycle. Endometriosis can be very painful due to scar tissue and adhesions, and it can inhibit fertility. This is one of the more physically painful conditions and can be aggravated by too much sugar in the diet. Unfortunately, with their doctors' grim prognoses, many women give up on the idea of having children naturally.

What's the Emotional Cause?

The reproductive organs are located within the sacral chakra, which is the energy center of relationships/sexuality, creativity, and children. The uterus and ovaries represent the point of creation. They're where creativity comes from, but also literally where life is created. Because of the areas the endometriosis surrounds, such as the uterus, ovaries (points of creation/femininity), and bowels (fear of letting go of what's no longer needed), this condition represents your creativity or ability to create being surrounded or strangled. Emotionally this manifests as hanging on to disappointment, frustration, and insecurity. It also often involves blaming the self or someone else. You want to look at the areas in your life that the sacral chakra represents: relationships (sexual or otherwise), creativity, and children. Which of these areas carries those negative feelings for you? This can be tough to explore because, as some of my clients have said, "Why would I purposely put myself in this much pain? I don't blame myself! I blame God, or this disease," etc. Because the physical condition is so painful, it can be hard to step back and look at the emotional cause objectively. I promise that there's something for you to look at. Remember, it's not about blaming yourself for "causing" the condition; it's your body giving you a check engine light, albeit a painful one.

The fact that we can shift our physical condition by shifting our thoughts is amazing and empowering. Give yourself the opportunity to step back and look into the Petri dish of your life and discover what might correlate based on these causes. See the following for a starting point.

What Can You Do About It?

Write down all of your responses to the following questions. The process of writing helps you sort things out.

- Go back to when you first noticed symptoms of endometriosis and inquire where you might have been hanging on to frustration, insecurity, or disappointment.

It's a learned pattern, not an innate one, which is good because that means we can shift it.

- Did family or friends let you down?

- Do you blame yourself for a parent leaving, and that's how you internalized it?

- Do you blame yourself or God for having a miscarriage?

- Did a significant other or family member abuse you?

- Have you not fully processed a breakup? Do you blame that person or yourself?

- Did you have a troubled relationship with a family member and you blame them for certain circumstances in your life?

- What isn't fair in your life?

- What do you feel is "surrounding" you (like the tissue surrounding your ability to create)?

Really do some deep inquiry here. Write as much as you can about each area and give yourself the time to sit with it. Feel how hurtful these issues are and see if you can decide to be done with them. Then take your list and burn it as a symbolic "I'm finished with this."

After you're done, write down three action steps you can take to move forward, such as doing belief sheets on the topics that came up in your brain dumps, writing about why the things that came up were actually purposeful, or treating your body to an hour of pampering (bodywork, massage, etc.). Then actually go do those things!

Basil and Geranium essential oils by Young Living can help with the pain as you're working through the mental and emotional causes.

You also might want to try a linden infusion (recipe is in the Conceivable Tool Kit). It really helps with the inflammation in the body and has been very helpful for my clients.

When you're dealing with a physical issue as painful as endometriosis, it can be difficult to step back and see a way out of it. Our brain has a tendency to think that because something has always been a certain way, it will continue to be, or to simply accept a care provider's verdict that we will never have children. You certainly can accept both of those mindsets, but know that I've had numerous cases of endometriosis disappear when my clients did some deep inquiry and processing.

My client Natalie had fibroids and endometriosis. In her case, the emotional cause was abuse and past partners not treating her well. She was scheduled to go in for surgery a couple of weeks after we started working together. We did some belief work and energy work. She really began to process some of her stuff in a way that she hadn't been able to before. When she went in for the surgery, they removed two fibroids (down from the eight she originally had), and the endometriosis was nowhere to be found. The doctors couldn't explain it. That is the power of doing this work. Clearing up our emotional baggage is key for moving our physical body forward.

8. Polycystic Ovarian Syndrome (PCOS)

As the name implies, polycystic ovarian syndrome is many cysts on an ovary, which can inhibit ovulation and is one of the leading physical causes of infertility. It involves the endocrine system, so the thyroid, pituitary gland, and hormones can be affected. Symptoms include prolonged or infrequent periods, excess hair growth, acne, and excess weight gain.

What's the Emotional Cause?

Again, the cause of this condition can be kind of hard to hear sometimes, and we can feel under attack; but keeping an open mind, see where this makes sense for you:

It can be an amplified version of ovarian cysts, as already discussed (nursing old hurts from relationships, past or current). If we haven't processed hurt or anger from a past relationship, or our current partner has done something that we haven't forgiven them for, it can fester at this point of creation.

The cause can also be a denial of femininity and usually guilt, shame, or fear around sexuality or the genitals. It can often stem from abuse, or from your *perception* of what you've been taught about sexuality and plugging that into your programming. Some of the clients I've seen with PCOS were raised with very strong religious beliefs—and talk, thoughts, or actions around the genitals, sex, or sensuality are seen as sinful. So many women push down these thoughts, which manifests physically as PCOS. It can also happen if some abuse or perceived abuse happened and the girl didn't know how to process it, so it was stored in her body this way. It often begins in the teen years when our thoughts and experiences about sex are being formed.

This syndrome can be the result of not fully processing a termination. Again, it's not that we would ever consciously punish ourselves, but the body does react to our thoughts, and things can fester over time. If there's hurt or guilt, it will manifest in the area where the situation happened.

PCOS can also manifest as little volcanoes of anger about a work situation, but more than likely it's anger toward a current or past partner.

Since the cysts form on the ovaries, which represent the point of creation, they can result when our creativity is compromised. For example, my client Victoria wanted to go to art school, but her traditional parents insisted she go to engineering school. She harbored resentment for compromising her creative soul to please her parents, and so the cysts formed.

What Can You Do About It?

Go back and look at what happened around the time you started noticing symptoms of PCOS. Really dig.

Was it an isolated incident or a belief that something was "wrong"?

What can you tell that version of you now? Maybe how you understand how she felt, why this journey has been purposeful, and why it's okay to release that. What do you understand about and empathize with the "you" of that time?

What can you let go of? What no longer serves you? Often we are hanging on to anger, judgment, feelings of being judged or not good enough, placing too much importance on what a partner said, etc.

Visualize the cysts being surrounded with light and shrinking while saying something like this: "It's safe to be feminine, and I release those beliefs that are no longer serving me," "This body is a beautiful gift. I embrace my sensuality, and my body functions the way it's meant to," or "I am balanced and calm and choose to be in the flow."

The thoughts that are causing this condition are more than likely subconscious, so we really want to praise our body and embrace all of it, from the cramps to the cycles to the sexuality. If we are subconsciously ashamed or blaming our body, how can it perform well?

Red clover infusion and linden infusion are super-helpful in terms of regulating all hormones and relieving inflammation. (Recipes are in the Conceivable Tool Kit.)

Also, Oregano, Release, and SARA essential oils from Young Living have benefited my clients with PCOS.

9. Male Infertility (Low Sperm Count, Motility, etc.)

Male infertility occurs in 7 percent of men and accounts for 40 to 50 percent of infertility. It can be diagnosed if there's low sperm production, abnormal sperm function/motility, or blockages that prevent the delivery of sperm. Health problems and lifestyle choices (including too much alcohol, soda, soy, and other foods) can play a role as well.

What's the Emotional Cause, and What Can You Do About It?

This is one of the trickier conditions for me to address when the woman is open to alternative methods and modalities but the man isn't. We have to be crafty about how we address it. *But* it's absolutely addressable.

I've found that male infertility is usually the result of one of four things:

1. The woman is the breadwinner and/or the more dominant personality.

   Some men are cool with this, but for some, it is a blow to their male ego. Their psyche still harbors that primitive belief system where they hunt and you watch the nest. As discussed in chapter 1 (external factor #3), men need to feel that they are contributing in a significant way to the family. If it can't be financially, see where else he can contribute (DIY projects, paying bills, taking out the trash, walking the dog). The key is to really communicate how helpful it is for you that he's doing these things. Not only will he be more likely to do them without being asked, but it will rev up his opinion of himself, therefore translating to his morphology.

2. He's not where he wants to be in his career.

 Is he in a job he hates? Is he not in the field he wants to be in? Does he secretly want to be something else when he grows up?

 Encourage him to open up and share his dreams. Explore the possibilities of an advanced certification or a class that will move him toward that goal, or encourage a hobby that he'll find fulfilling so his life is not just about the job. Your support will go a long way. Just as it is important that you be in your purpose rather than just a job, the same is equally true for him. If he is an insurance broker but really wants to work with animals, you must start helping him lay the groundwork, because he won't do it on his own. He won't even think of it as a real option. The two of you being lit up and filled with purpose *is* part of getting the baby here. It's not taking time away from baby making, it's literally helping to make that a reality. Don't skip over this part.

3. He has unresolved family issues.

 Did one parent leave when he was younger? Did his parents get divorced, leaving him with unresolved guilt, sadness, and fear? Is he afraid of making a family because he doesn't want that to happen to his children? It would be great if you could have a conversation with him about his concerns or encourage him to speak to someone about them. If he's not up for that, see if he'd try acupuncture. It's a little more mainstream than this work, and it's not something he would have to bare his soul for. But it can reset his energy without him even realizing it.

4. He has financial fears.

 This is pretty self-explanatory. Kids cost money, and he may have doubts about being able to provide for this munchkin. Whether the fears are founded in reality or not, it's certainly important to reassure him. There's the old saying "If we wait until we're more financially ready, we'll never have a kid." It's so true. There will always be a reason to delay. He'll always feel like he's not quite there yet. Remind him that sometimes you just have to leap, trusting the Universe to provide what you need when you need it.

Meet with a financial advisor, or if you're good with money, break down for him how it could actually be okay financially. It is helpful for his brain to feel like you have a plan and that everything will work itself out.

Approach this from a heart-cracked-open place of "Hey, I totally get why you're scared. I feel that too, but here's some stuff I've figured out." It can help put him, and therefore his body, at ease.

I've also found that Idaho Blue Spruce essential oil by Young Living dabbed on his ankles and the base of his spine or Valor essential oil on his feet and the base of his spine work well if he's open to alternative suggestions. It can be done at night so he doesn't have to worry about smelling woodsy!

If it's your partner and not you who's dealing with the fertility component, it can seem a little hopeless. But there are things you can do to move him forward. My client Chloe's husband was dealing with low sperm count and motility. She was freaking out because she didn't see how she could help the situation. He was in an unfulfilling job that he couldn't shift at the time. Unbeknownst to him, she placed a piece of ruby-in-zoisite under his side of the bed. It's a good fertility stone for both men and women. Stones are also conductors. They absorb energy and, luckily for us, can absorb some of our "yuck." See the Stones and Crystals for Fertility 101 worksheet in the Conceivable Tool Kit to learn more about how they can be helpful in the fertility process for you and your partner.

Chloe would also casually put her hand over her husband's heart every night in bed and think, *I love you, you're safe, and we can do this*. Eventually he began to feel calmer and didn't feel the need to drink as much beer, which, as we discussed in chapter 1, can decimate sperm count. And *poof*! Pregnant! Incidentally, Chloe's husband has been *so* fulfilled that they got pregnant again right before their baby turned one! This is just another example of how any condition can be changed by shifting your thought process.

The important thing to realize is that if your partner is going through this, it's an opportunity for you to put your desire for a baby aside for a minute and focus on reconnecting with your partner. You guys are a team first and foremost. And you want to make sure your teammate is okay and that you're giving him the best support possible so that he can be the best possible version of himself. Try to resist the urge to shuffle him through this process as fast as possible so that you can get to the baby. Date each other. Connect to each other. Believe in each other.

10. Unexplained Infertility

As the name implies, doctors can't find a cause of infertility in these cases. This situation can be most enigmatic and frustrating. Because there is no clear problem, there is no clear solution. Many of my clients have said they almost wish they had a "legit" physical condition because they feel it would be easier to treat.

A myriad of factors can contribute to unexplained infertility, but I guarantee that it's not because you had that cup of coffee or aren't eating enough kale. Yes, it's important to eat as clean as possible, but that's not *the* reason you're not getting pregnant. Sometimes we obsess about eating the right food and the right amount of it, and that can feed into our Type-A-ness and exacerbate the situation. Remember, there are people who don't take care of themselves but are still able to get pregnant, so don't go too crazy about the food component.

What's the Emotional Cause, and What Can You Do About It?

See if you are plugging into one or more beliefs that aren't true, such as "I'm running out of time. I'm too old. I'm gonna be an old mom and die before my kid graduates high school. It should have happened by now. It was easy for my friend, so it should be easy for me," and so on. If any of these sting, do a belief sheet on it so you can free up that energy to move forward.

Do you have fear around the birth process itself? That's pretty common. The way birth is portrayed in the movies is scary, and many women we know have had traumatic births, so we think we will too. Even when women relay their normal birth stories, it can sound terrifying. So can the process of being pregnant, for that matter. Hemorrhoids? Gas? Constipation? Losing control of your bowels during labor? Yikes! If your brain/ego thinks labor is scary and disgusting and you might die, it will try to do you a solid and just avoid the whole situation. We want to find ways to become comfortable with the idea of birth and believe that the process can actually be beautiful rather than scary. To build your confidence around the idea of birth and actually get excited about it, look at the 2008 documentary *The Business of Being Born* and the book *Ina May's Guide to Childbirth*. I'd also recommend attending a doula or HypnoBirthing workshop. Even if you don't want to teach or become certified in either of these modalities, they do an amazing job of helping you see birth as the amazing, empowering experience it's meant to be. Watch HypnoBirthing videos on YouTube to see how calm, beautiful, and empowering the birth process can be.

Do you have any unresolved anxiety, body issues/eating disorders, or family issues? Do a brain dump, and list all of the things that come up, no matter how stupid or frivolous they sound. Circle the top three things that feel gross to you and do a belief sheet on them. If you harbor ongoing or unresolved issues, find someone to help you process them and allow your body to resume normal functioning.

Refer again to the list of fifteen external factors affecting fertility in chapter 1. These are often the reasons for unexplained infertility, especially having a stressful job and being a super planner. We'll go more into the energy of why those things are not helpful in chapter 4.

When dealing with all of these issues, we will be tempted to say, "I'll fix it once I'm pregnant." Fix it now. Address what you can to get your energy moving forward.

This is where your automatic fight-or-flight response is getting triggered big time. Remember that when you have these stressors, whether they be external factors or internal beliefs, your body goes into survival mode. And since you don't need your reproductive system when you're about to fight or take flight from a situation, it slows or shuts down. If you are in the unexplained fertility category, I guarantee you that your brain is triggered about something. It might not be super-obvious to you, because rationally you're pretty sure this isn't going to kill you. But your primal brain doesn't know that—and that's who we have to convince. We can't shut off this response just because we want to. There is no fooling the brain. So we have to really investigate what's triggering it and figure out how we can create space and a feeling of capability in our life. Taking a deep dive into these things may seem invasive to your brain, but I promise you, it's way less invasive and way less expensive than IVF.

Your body is waiting for you to trust it to do what women have done for millennia, what you were built to do. Unfortunately, so many of us connect to the fear of friends and family who had a hard time getting pregnant. Then we are fed dire announcements by media and doctors that once you hit thirty, getting pregnant is going to be hard, and even if you do conceive, your body's a ticking time bomb that will produce a deformed baby, or you may die in childbirth. While I'm sure the people who tell us these things have the best of intentions, fear is instilled in us early on. As a result, we stop trusting our intuition and our bodies and start trusting someone who barely knows us to tell us what we are capable of.

We tend to give up all of our power to the doctors, to the condition, to the fear of what could be. You have much more power on this journey that you realize, and examining this condition from a different perspective is just one way to take back that power. Going inward to inquire and listen to your intuition will serve you immensely on this journey.

Nobody knows your body better than you. You just have to remember to plug in and hear what your body is telling you. Use a mantra like "I trust you" over and over, with your eyes closed and a hand on your belly. That would be a great daily practice. You and your body are on the same team. See if you can listen to what it's telling you.

4

Manifesting Your Munchkin

Why where you're putting your energy matters

This is perhaps the most important part of the book. We're going to be talking about the Law of Attraction as it applies to fertility, the idea that where you're putting your energy matters. This is where the common pitfalls can show up.

Many of us have heard about the Law of Attraction through the movie or book *The Secret*. We think that all of a sudden we can wield this "secret" to instantaneously realize our dreams. We learn how to hunker down, think positive, focus on what we want (or so we think), and yet, we still don't have a baby. So we try harder, read more books, focus more ... and the baby still isn't coming.

There are a lot more nuances to this Law of Attraction than we realize. My clients who are smart, driven women *think* they're taking the right steps and *think* they're being positive. But the truth is that most of them aren't (and they have zero clue). So it's vital to understand what's really happening so you can take charge and effect a powerful shift.

Unfortunately, what most of us get from preliminary Law of Attraction exposure is that if we focus *really, really* hard and we *really, really* want it, the Universe will deliver a baby (or a car or a million dollars, etc.).

Here's the problem:

The Law of Attraction means that like energy attracts like energy. Essentially, whatever energy you're putting out, the Universe answers by handing you a situation that's an energetic match. What we focus on we get more of.

One of the biggest pitfalls with the Law of Attraction is *attachment*, which we started to talk about in the belief work in chapter 2. When we first start working with the Law of Attraction, we're taught that what we think about we bring about. So we believe that if we think about nothing else 24/7, a baby will materialize. This is when we're *really* focused on what we want, almost to the point of obsession.

Here's why that's not helpful:

Like energy attracts like energy, right? So if you're putting out "I *need* to be pregnant, I *have* to be a mother, I'll *make* myself pregnant," the Universe is hearing the lack. "Need" means you don't have. "Have to" means you need it and are forcing it. I'll "make it happen" means it hasn't happened yet and something is wrong, and also that you don't trust the Universe because you are taking "control."

So while we *think* we're being positive, we're really mired in the desperate, needing, forcing energy that's just attracting more of the same.

A good way to know if you're attached to something is if you put conditions on your energy. *If it's conditional, you're attached.* If you say, "I'm being positive so I can have the baby," or "I'll let my guard down with my mother if she'll let hers down with me," or "I'm putting my energy into feeling like I'm pregnant, so I better not get my period," you're attached.

We want to feel these positive things because they feel good and (via the Law of Attraction) can bring more good. We know we haven't truly put *all* of our energy into it when there's a condition attached.

Whatever is happening in our life, we've attracted it—positive or negative. We choose it not consciously but energetically. That's a tough pill to swallow for a lot people, myself included when I started this work. I cried, "What do you *mean* I'm attracting debt into my life? Of course I don't want it!"

But that was the problem. I was so focused on the fact that I was in debt and scared because I didn't have enough money (which was a belief, and that belief work we talked about in chapter 2 helped me) that I couldn't help but attract more of "being in debt." The cycle continued until I started choosing thoughts that felt good to me, such as "I do have enough money for _____. I make enough money to enjoy life (versus survive it). I am supported by the Universe."

So we need to focus on what we *do* want versus what we *don't* want. As humans, we tend to focus on the problem, not the solution, and that keeps our wheels spinning. It's like a broken record: "I'm never going to get pregnant, I'm never going to get pregnant, I'm never going to get pregnant." That message will keep repeating until you lift the arm of the record player and put it on a different track. There has to be a conscious choice to change the track.

You may say, "Well, if I could change it, I would." Know that's a belief. That's your brain kicking in wanting to be right. The future isn't set and neither is the present, which is *so awesome*!

It can be overwhelming to know that we have a responsibility for what happens in our life, but I want to get you excited about the fact that *you're responsible*. Because that means if your life isn't going how you want, you get to change it—and that's *so* empowering. It takes us out of the victim place (this happened *to* me) and puts us in the empowered place (this happened *for* me).

Remember from our belief work in chapter 2 that everything that's happening in our life *should* be happening because it *is* happening. Whether "good" or "bad," it's happening because there's something we're supposed to learn from it. That lesson will keep coming up throughout your life until you address it. Patterns like money issues, dating the wrong type of guy, dead-end careers, multiple miscarriages, and not being able to get pregnant are not permanent issues. It feels like it because they keep coming up, but they keep coming up because we haven't dealt with the energetic pattern. When that is addressed, you won't be an energetic match to the pattern anymore and it won't ever show up in your life again.

So when you notice things in your life that you'd like to be different, can you approach it from an exploratory place of "Huh. This is not what I want in my life right now, but it's happening because it's supposed to show me something to work on. What could that be? What changes can I make, who can I forgive, what beliefs no longer serve me?"

Your life won't change because you *say* you want it to. It will change when you consciously direct your energy toward what you want versus what you don't want. You already know what you don't want. No need to spend more wheel-spinning time there.

Look at your list of external factors from chapter 1. I bet you could make some tweaks there. Read the belief material in chapter 2 again. It's therapy on crack when you dig enough, and I would venture to say that it's the most important piece in my work with clients.

This process is what I call ERA: Excavation, Realization, Action. We need to excavate from your subconscious those things that are holding back the baby's arrival. We need to bring your awareness to the issue and realize that these are thoughts, and thoughts can be changed. Then you can take action to move through them, whether through daily meditation, grounding, belief sheets, making a list of what you're most looking forward to when you're pregnant (that you look at every day), making space in your dwelling (and your schedule) for this baby, etc.

It's hard when the thing you want most feels out of your grasp and you really want to reach it. The more you reach for it, the more it runs away, so you reach more and it runs even further away. So instead of hunting it, set out some bait (in a non-manipulative way, of course) and lure it to you. That way you're not wasting any energy going after it.

> Hunting it says: "I *need* you to survive and if I don't have you I'm gonna die [which is honestly how it can feel to your brain]. *If I can't be a mother, I'm gonna die.*"

> Putting out the bait says: "I'm giving you what you want, and you can give me what I want. I *invite* you in when you're ready. In the meantime I'm aligning myself with thoughts and things that fill me up, light me up," and so on. It's being in a state of allowing.

Think about those two different energies for a second:

> Hunting: "I need this baby to come. If I can't be a mother, my life is pointless. I need you, baby. Where are you? Why won't you come?"

> Allowing: "I invite the next step. I'm making this warm, cozy place for you to hang out in. I'm being good to my body and releasing beliefs that no longer serve me. I'm making space for you, and I'm so looking forward to meeting you. I'm excited for the moment the midwife hands you to me and I look in your eyes for the first time. I'm ready, baby, and I invite you in when you're ready."

It takes a lot of energy to be in the "hunting" energy. It's exhausting just saying those words and feeling that energy for a few seconds, let alone residing in that place most of the time. I immediately felt relaxation and excitement with the second one, and it tapped into my knowing that I am capable of what women before me and around me are capable of.

Allowing feels much easier energy-wise. We're taught that life is hard, and when we've experienced difficulty getting pregnant, we think it's an

uphill battle. Many of us are taught that the harder we work for something, the more worthwhile it is. But according to the Law of Attraction,
it's closer to "The harder you try... the harder you try." Like energy
attracts like energy, so if we're putting out the energy that pregnancy is
an uphill battle that might not succeed, then the Universe hears, "Cue
Mount Everest and an avalanche!"

So how do we get unattached? First, know that if you're attached,
you're not in your intuition; you're in your brain. Your intuition knows
everything is, and will be, fine. Your brain, however, is freaked out and
thinks the apocalypse is near. Remember, the brain needs to keep you alive,
and when you want to go down an unfamiliar path, the flight-or-flight
response is triggered because your brain isn't entirely sure it will survive.

The next thing you want to do is get into a grounding routine. As
I said in chapter 2, most of us are driving our body around from our
head. So we want to do things that get us back in our body, such as the
following:

- Yoga

- A five-minute meditation where you put a hand on your
  belly, close your eyes, and invite the baby's energy in

- Dancing in your living room to some kick-ass music

- Being in nature for at least a few minutes as you connect to
  the ground. Release the crap that's not serving you into the
  ground and then draw up power from the earth to recharge
  yourself.

- Listening to inspirational music as you take deep breaths in
  through your nose and exhale deeply through your mouth,
  focusing only on your breath.

- Knitting or some other sort of activity with your hands

- Taking deep breaths as your hands and feet connect to the ground

- Taking a belly dancing or pole dancing class

- Taking a bath with essential oils

- Going for a walk in your neighborhood (preferably in nature)

- Working out—cardio or strength training

These are all ways to get you more plugged into your intuition. Also take an inventory of what you believe about getting pregnant. Look again at the list in chapter 2 of the ten most common beliefs women struggling with fertility are plugged into, and see if they resonate. Then run them through a belief sheet. As a reminder, we want to get down and dirty, petty and scared, and feel the emotions that come up so that at the turn-arounds we can let go of them. Do you feel like you're running out of time? Do you fear that you'll have another miscarriage because you've had one before? Do you feel you should have been pregnant by now?

Nip these beliefs in the bud, because they will permeate the rest of your journey until they're addressed. Once the attachment is gone, we're no longer pulling in that desperate energy because we're trusting that everything is happening the way it's supposed to be happening. We start pulling in a calmer energy and we're able to take action and move forward from where we *are* rather than wishing the situation were different from what it is. We can wish it were different all day long, but the fact is, it's not. See if you can explore why and then take steps to move forward from a neutral position.

Start from "This is where I am right now. It's not where I want to be, but it's what *is* right now. What are some ways I can move forward?" That takes much less energy than "I should be pregnant by now, I should be pregnant by now."

When you notice yourself getting frustrated with this process, take a step back and find where you're investing your energy. Are you putting it toward what you don't want (the problem) or what you do want (the solution)?

Hint: If it's stressing you out, it's the problem. Let's find a way to reframe it in a positive light so we can begin pulling the positive-solution energy toward us, thereby changing our current circumstances to what we want.

Here are two examples of things that need reframing:

We're trying to get pregnant. Remember, like energy attracts like energy, so trying brings more trying or more "not quite" there energy. Reframe it to something like "We've started the process of expanding our family" or "We are making space for a new addition."

The week of my period. When you refer to the first three weeks of the month as trying and the last as the week of your period, where is the room for the baby? "The week of my period" says to the Universe that you're expecting your period. Many of my clients' energy totally shifts to fear that week because they are deathly afraid they're going to get their period, and when you're looking for your period to show up, the Universe has to answer with like energy and bring it to you. Let's reframe *period week* as *testing week:* "This will be the week where I get to test!" Make the wallpaper on your phone a picture of a positive pregnancy test. Every time you see it, imagine how awesome it's going to feel when you see that positive sign. How will you tell your husband/partner? Even when you consciously stop noticing the picture, subconsciously you're still thinking, "Yeah, it *is* going to be awesome *when* that happens."

Another pitfall with the Law of Attraction is that the experts say to phrase it "as if it has already happened." In a lot of cases that can work, but in the case of fertility it's hard for a lot of people to say "I'm pregnant" when they're not, or "I have a baby" when they don't. It kind of feels like "F★★★ you, I don't, and this isn't helping!" Feeling this frustration makes it easy to disconnect from the idea of manifesting at all because our brain just isn't having it. It's too big of an energetic gap to go from a hard fertility journey to being pregnant.

My clients find it helpful to say, "It's going to be awesome *when* ____."

You've had awesome things happen to you in the past (I would hope!). You know what excitement and goose bumps feel like. You know how much you're looking forward to seeing that heartbeat on the sonogram or registering for baby gifts or hearing that first cry.

That's something you can plug into on a feeling level, and *that's* the key to all of this. You can think stuff all day long, and it won't happen. It's when you *feel* it that things begin to shift on a cellular level. And we can't be in attachment when we're feeling these positive things. Energetically you can't be in excitement and hopelessness at the same time.

One of my clients wrote her baby a song, which helped her get out of her head and into her body, where she could tune in to the energy of her baby coming. She also made a list of everything she was looking forward to, down to the most inane thing, and hung it everywhere (like the picture of the positive pregnancy test I mentioned). Your brain is continually seeing "It's gonna be awesome when ____," and the Universe goes, "Yeah, it *is* gonna be awesome. Here's some awesome." That list, when you really *feel* into each item (eyes closed, hand on your heart, dropping into your body), not only helps you be clear to the Universe about what you want, it also puts *out* the energy you're actually wanting *back*.

So often on this journey we become so focused on what's going wrong. We're frustrated with our bodies, we're annoyed with people who keep asking when we're having kids, and we're constantly trying to push down the dread, desperation, and "need" that we might not be able to be a mom.

The problem with that is that from a Law of Attraction perspective, like energy attracts like energy. The Universe doesn't respond to what you're *saying*, it responds to the *energy* you're putting out. You can say "I really, really, really want to be a mom. I'm going to *make* it happen." But if the energy underneath is "Oh god, what if it doesn't happen? I'm so scared it's not going to happen," then *that's* the energy you're being met with.

It's not our fault. It's how we're taught to think. We focus on the problem, not the solution, and most of us are not aware of where we are placing our thoughts and energy. But if you want things to shift, you have to start becoming aware.

You want to bring the focus to what you're *excited* about in this journey. Being excited brings things to be excited about. So write things that, when they happen, you will be overjoyed at. Notice I said *when*, not *if*. You must get in the mindset that this is going to happen—that you're *expecting* it.

Once you've written down all of these things, take each one individually and close your eyes, with a hand on your heart. Take a deep breath and say the first thing three times. *Feel* what happens in your body—notice what happens when you really let yourself get absorbed in a thought such as *when I walk back into the bathroom and see the positive sign on the pregnancy test*. What do you notice? Chills? Can't stop smiling? Can't stop crying? Feel it all. That's when things begin to change on a cellular level.

For things to really start changing, you must align with what you *want* versus what you *don't* want. Many of my clients are afraid to do this exercise because they feel like they'll be more disappointed or that it will hurt more if it doesn't work out. There are a lot of nuances to this manifesting/positivity thing. You can't "hope" it's going to work. Hope says "I really want it, but I'm really scared it won't work." That's when the disappointment sets in—because your energy is split. On-the-fence energy brings on-the-fence results. So we must work on being brave enough

to be open and allow ourselves to feel joy and excitement around pregnancy, because the Law of Attraction is a faithful friend: if you put out
joy and excitement, that's what you will get back. So let's dive in.

Make a list of twenty items starting with "It's going to be awesome
when_____." (You'll find the It's Going to Be Awesome When worksheet in the Conceivable Tool Kit.)

Our ninety-miles-an-hour brains want to *think* everything. Take
time daily to sit with that list and *feel* into the awesomeness of it without being scared that it won't happen. The coolest thing about the Law
of Attraction is that when you commit your energy to cracking open
and receiving, you can't *not* get what you want. It's that tricky sliver of
scared, stuck energy hanging back that keeps us in the same place. A
part of you says, "I don't want to put all my eggs in one basket, because
then I won't be as disappointed." But that's actually the problem. That
sliver of energy that's hanging back out of self-preservation is the thing
that's actually holding you back. It's the thing that causes the tentative,
mediocre results. When you are energetically on the fence about something, you don't get real results—certainly not the ones that you want.
We actually want to say to the Universe, "Here's my basket of eggs! I'm
all in and I'm excited about it!"

Think of it as deciding to change lanes. If you're driving in the right
lane and you keep running into things you don't like, you're going to
keep running into them unless you decide to put your turn signal on
and move into the left lane. When you do, you're not aligned with the
cars in the right lane anymore. If you're aligned with what you want,
then what you don't want can't vibrate in the same space.

You can't *hope* it'll happen. Hope means we're leaving it up to the
thing in the sky, or that there's something out there that decides whether
or not we can have our dream. Remember that you are co-creating your
life, whether you realize it or not. You have orchestrated every experience that comes into your life, so *choose* what you want.

Those of you who've read Esther Hicks's books might know about the three steps to creation: ask, believe, receive. *Ask* the Universe for what you want. *Believe* it can happen. *Receive* it.

It's not our job to know *how* it's going to happen or *when* it's going to happen. That's the Universe's job. Our job is to focus on the *what*, to trust and feel into what we would love. Giving up that degree of control is great because it takes so much pressure off us not to have to figure out the details.

I want to share with you a couple examples of my clients putting the Law of Attraction into practice.

My client Gemma had two miscarriages and was convinced she'd have another one. We did a lot of belief work and energy work around that, and she did get pregnant! But around week seven, she started spotting and understandably freaked out. This was the time when the other miscarriages had started. She couldn't help but think it was happening again, and it was very likely, so we had to turn her energy around *fast*. I asked her, "If you couldn't think the thought that it was happening again, what would you think about instead?

She answered, "Spotting is normal in the first trimester." She took a deep breath and felt into that. She felt it in her bones that it was normal and everything was fine. She got herself into her body, where she could access her intuition, and out of her head, where her brain was having a field day convincing her that she was about to have another miscarriage. At that moment she took the reins and changed what she didn't want into what she did want. She reminded herself of her victories and how much she deserved this. She stopped that miscarriage from happening and gave birth in January. She *believed* it, and that's the key. If she'd stayed in the fear, she very likely would have lost the baby. She took control of her power and did it—and you can too.

My client Jenny was having a hard time getting pregnant. She had tried nutritional counseling, acupuncture, and fertility treatments, but nothing was working. Her main beliefs were "It should have happened by now" and "It's not going to happen." We realized that she was so overwhelmed between moving, her and her husband starting new jobs, and this pervasive anxiety that it might not happen that she was in kind of an energetic holding pattern. After working through some of these beliefs, she really focused on the reasons why she *would* be pregnant and also got to the point where she stepped back from the fear and said, "I'm choosing the baby over the fear." Her anxiety was almost debilitating, but she was so ready to be done with being ruled by fear that she was able to gather her energy and direct it toward the baby. Now she's no longer dealing with debilitating levels of anxiety, and with all the energy she gathered, she gave birth to twins!

So just know that these women are no different from you in terms of their capability to manifest. You can change any physical condition by changing your thought patterns.

Besides getting pregnant, my clients have done the following:

- Shrunk ovarian cysts

- Reversed hypothyroidism naturally

- Stopped a miscarriage

- Released scar tissue naturally

- Doubled their uterine lining

- Tripled the number of follicles

- Repaired relationships

- Healed male infertility

- Processed grief over past losses or terminations

- Healed endometriosis

You can choose the pregnancy over the fear. *Acknowledging and embracing that you have a choice is key.* That can be hard to hear because you already feel like you've *been* choosing. But it's been coming from a place of lack and desperation. Armed with the knowledge of how to shift your energy, challenge yourself to commit your energy to what you'd love instead of what you're afraid you'll never have. It makes all the difference. You're the only one who can do that for yourself. But that's the awesome thing: *You. Can. Shift. This.* You can decide to lift the arm of the record player and put it on a new track.

Where you're putting your energy matters, so lean toward what you want (deciding) versus what you don't want (attachment). It can be tricky walking that fine line between choosing and attachment because they sound similar, but energetically they're very different. Sometimes we can catch it and sometimes we need an outside eye to flag what we're missing because we can't see our own shit. This book is one part of the work I do, and I hope you've gotten some insights and tools to get you on your way to your little munchkin.

5

....

Chakras

What they represent and how they relate to fertility

Chakras are energy centers in the body. The word *chakra* comes from the Sanskrit word meaning "wheel" or "turning wheel." These energy centers spin like wheels. There are many chakras throughout the body, but there are seven main ones that go from the base of the spine to the top of the head. They all represent different things, and when I'm working with my clients, if I notice that a certain chakra is closed or not spinning, it gives me an idea of where she might be blocked. Blocked energy can lead to illness, the body not functioning as it's meant to, and feeling powerless and disconnected.

As we discuss the seven chakras and their meanings, I'll give you some tips on how to open them up so that your energy is functioning at an optimum level.

Root Chakra

Color: Red
Represents: Grounding, family, knowing who you are, finances, etc.
Location: Base of the spine

Sacral Chakra

Color: Orange
Represents: Sexuality, relationships, creativity, children
Location: Lower abdomen

Solar Plexus Chakra

Color: Yellow
Represents: Your power center, drive, ambition, confidence
Location: Upper abdomen

Heart Chakra

Color: Green
Represents: Love and inner peace, the most "you" place you can be
Location: Chest

Throat Chakra

Color: Blue
Represents: Voicing your opinion, feeling like you're being heard, expressing your feelings and truth
Location: Throat

Third Eye Chakra

Color: Indigo
Represents: Intuition, wisdom, imagination, ability to zoom out and see the bigger picture
Location: Middle of the forehead

Crown Chakra

Color: Purple
Represents: Spiritual/universe-y awareness, connection to Source
Location: Top of the head

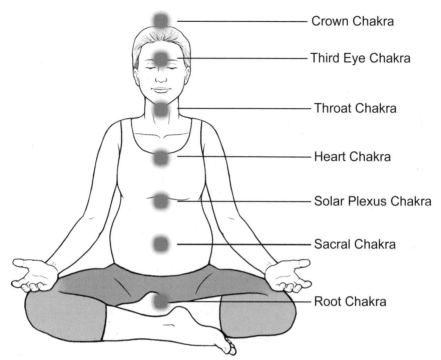

The Seven Main Chakras

Let's explore how these chakras and their meanings can relate to fertility, and how you can use them to aid you in moving toward getting your little munchkin here.

Root Chakra

The root chakra can be closed for a few reasons. When dealing with infertility, we are often spending way more time in our head than in our body. If you are a super Type-A, analytical, overscheduled, cerebral person struggling with OCD, there's a good chance your root chakra is closed. It can also be closed if you're having a hard time with family members, if you're worried about money, or if there's been some chaos in your life and you're not feeling grounded. The root chakra is about feeling safe, and on this fertility journey there are so many unknowns that it's hard to feel safe.

I know these things may not seem related to fertility, but for us to overcome our challenges, we must feel that we are grounded and on a steady enough foundation to build this thing that we want. If the root chakra is closed, it's also just a wonderful indicator that you need to create more space in your life, whether it's releasing beliefs that aren't serving you anymore or finding places to make room in your insane schedule. As I mentioned earlier, if your brain feels like you are stretched too thin, it will send the signal to your reproductive system that it's not going to add yet another thing for you to take care of.

A good first step is to establish a daily grounding routine. It doesn't have to be for a long time—ten to fifteen minutes per day would be fantastic. Find an activity that gets you into your body, where you don't have to think about or analyze anything and your body feels really safe and grounded. Here are some good grounding activities:

- Yoga

- Meditation

- Guided meditation

- Dancing in the living room to your favorite jams

- Taking a bath with your favorite essential oil

- Going for a walk

- Sitting in nature for a few minutes (preferably with hands and feet touching the ground)

- Knitting or doing some mindless activity with your hands

- Bodywork (massage, reiki, acupuncture, etc.)

- Nourishing herbal infusions

It's important that the root chakra is open so we feel safe to carry on with this journey that our brain is scared of, and we have a solid foundation to build our dreams on.

Sacral Chakra

The sacral chakra can be closed for a couple of different reasons. Relationships, creativity, and children are all related to this chakra, so if you're having or have had problems in one or more of these areas, the others will be affected as well.

Here are some of the most common things I see with my clients whose sacral chakra is closed or not spinning: endometriosis, fibroids, cysts, and PCOS (polycystic ovary syndrome) due to hurt or blame from past relationships that is now manifesting in the body. A lot of this is, of course, subconscious, but when there are things we haven't processed from past hurts, it can lead to a closed sacral chakra and delay the arrival of the munchkin.

If you are a creative person but are not using these skills, this energy center can be closed. If you're an artist working in corporate America, a chef working as an accountant, or a life coach working as a professor, this is an issue. There's nothing wrong with any of these careers; it's more that if you're on the planet to be an artist and you're not doing that, then this area can suffer. It doesn't always have to be that you make it your career; but if you enjoy gardening, painting, or singing and you don't make time for it, the sacral chakra can slow down or stop spinning. Just like with relationships, this can affect the baby's timing.

There are some big things to be processed and healed here, so it's important that you don't try to gloss over it. What are some action steps you can take to move forward from this?

- Sign up for voice lessons (or the equivalent for your creative thing)
- Block off some time this weekend to garden

- Do some belief work on the relationships in your life that are hurtful

- Do some visualizations (filling the area with light, shrinking the fibroids, etc.)

- With a hand on your abdomen, visualize an orange orb spinning in that area. See it glowing bigger and brighter and spinning faster. Then see if you can connect to the energy of the baby. Just observe and see if you get a feeling, a visual, or something that confirms your connection to the baby. Building that connection is important so that you feel there is someone there for you, versus a blob in the ether who may or may not arrive.

Solar Plexus Chakra

For the solar plexus chakra, our drive and ambition center, I usually find that my clients are having an issue in the work arena if this area is closed. As I mentioned earlier, career and fertility are tightly linked. We have to feel confident, capable, and in our purpose to succeed at work, and feel confident and capable in ourselves to make a baby. The solar plexus is our power center, and if we're not feeling powerful in our lives, it makes it much more difficult to move forward and achieve the things we want most.

Most people are not being "what they want to be when they grow up." They are in a job they feel obligated to be in versus something that really lights them up every day. Most often this is a result of being influenced by parents who direct them into what is an "acceptable" career, or they want a certain lifestyle and think that there are only certain jobs that will pay them enough money, so they sacrifice their purpose for a paycheck. This is not a judgment at all. It's a survival mechanism. It makes sense that we would do that. I am finding, though, that there's a big energetic shift going on in the world. More and more we are called to be in our purpose versus just a job. When we ignore our purpose, the other areas in our life are often not in alignment or we're not able to make progress. Here are some steps you can take to open your solar plexus chakra:

- Put a citrine crystal on your solar plexus when you're meditating. It helps with resolving work issues, building confidence, and opening your solar plexus.

- Visualize a yellow orb spinning at your solar plexus. See it getting bigger and brighter and spinning faster. This can be done at any time—while meditating, during your lunch break, before you get out of bed, etc. It only takes about a minute, but it can really help open this energy center.

- Let yourself dream about what you'd really love to be doing, even if you have no idea how it would happen. Write down what you'd love. What would make you feel powerful? Take some time to sit in the feeling of how awesome that will be.

If you are aligned in the career area, the fertility area (and others) will follow. Align yourself with what you want versus what you don't want, and summon your innate strength and capability.

Heart Chakra

The heart chakra represents joy, love, and peace. If this area is closed, it's likely due to a loss (such as a miscarriage or a death in the family) or giving up on yourself.

If you've had a loved one pass away in the last few years, that can be affecting your ability to allow in joy and love, because your heart is still sad and processing the grief. If you've endured one or more miscarriages, the heart chakra can be closed because of the pain of the loss and the fear that it may never work out, and because your body doesn't want to be hurt anymore. So this energy center shuts down to preserve the self. Also, if this has been a long journey for you, this energy center can be closed if you've started to lose hope. Here are some things you can do to open the heart chakra:

- Get a green aventurine or green calcite stone. Place it on your heart when you're meditating. You can even wear it in your bra!

- Visualize a green orb spinning at your heart. See it getting bigger and brighter and spinning faster.

- If you've lost a loved one or had a miscarriage, connect to them. You can do this by writing a letter or journal entry to the person. You can also do it through visualization: close your eyes, picture them there with you, and say and feel everything you need to. It's important to feel these things and then choose to let them go. Ask the person's spirit/energy to help you move forward, and see if you can release some of the grief that's not serving you.

Often when something traumatic happens, we try to move through it as quickly as possible as a survival mechanism. We may consciously think we've processed these things, but we really haven't. We don't like feeling this stuff, so we try to hurry up and get through it. But if your heart is closed off, you're being called to really feel this stuff, to sit in being uncomfortable, to move through it, and then to choose to let it go.

Throat Chakra

The throat chakra is a really important one in fertility. It represents the ability to voice your opinion, to be yourself, and to feel you're being heard. As mentioned in chapter 3, if there's a thyroid issue connected to this chakra, it can be the result of humiliation, not being able to speak up, or wondering "When's it going to be my turn?" For some women this area is blocked due to poor communication with their spouse, and not being able to fully be themselves and say what they need to say. For some it's an issue with a boss or coworkers at their job, and they're unable to voice their opinions or feel heard. And for others it's related to their families. If they come from a tight-knit or culturally strong family, they can feel judged by family members and communication can be compromised. So what can you do to open the throat chakra?

- Use a blue kyanite stone, which is helpful for learning to voice things in a way where people hear you and for finding the courage to speak. Place it on your throat while meditating, and carry it on your person when encountering one of those people who make you feel that you can't voice your opinion. Set the intention for the stone to help open the lines of communication in a way that is beneficial for all.

- With eyes closed, visualize a blue orb spinning at your throat. See it getting bigger and brighter and spinning faster and faster. Keep doing this until the orb extends to about a foot outside your body, all the while spinning. This will help keep that area open.

- Write a brain dump about how your voice is being stifled and by whom. Notice what fears or judgments come up, and try doing a belief sheet from chapter 2.

- What are three steps you can take to exercise your voice from an empowered place rather than a forceful one? They don't have to be huge things to start, but commit to these three things. This will go a long way toward shifting your energy.

- Sing. Get that area of your body used to vocalizing and projecting.

It may not seem like the throat is related to fertility, but when the throat chakra is closed or compromised, it can be a problem. Your body feels safer when it feels it can speak and be heard. If your brain thinks you're not being heard, the last thing it wants to do is add another thing to your plate—another place where someone else's voice will matter more than yours. While this is a block to fertility, don't just work on it to get the baby. This has probably been a pattern in your life for a while, and it's important for your overall life (and not just the baby) that you address this. You must make sure you're being heard. No one else will.

Third Eye Chakra

The third eye (or brow) chakra is at your forehead. It represents your intu- ition center, clear thinking, and that "knowing" when something is true or not. It's very common for this chakra to be blocked because most of us are in our heads so much of the time. This is especially the case if we tend to be of the Type-A persuasion. Our brain/ego runs the show most of the time, and many of us are too busy analyzing things down to a bloody stump to pay attention to our intuition. If we are anxious or in a fight-or- flight state, our brain will come up with all kinds of crazy, scary scenarios that just keep our wheels spinning. But if we can find a way to operate from our intuition, we don't question our decisions and we are able to feel what the best course of action is. So how can we open this chakra?

- Use an amethyst or moonstone on your forehead when you meditate. Both of these are for opening your intuition center. If stones aren't your thing, place one of your hands on your forehead and breathe deeply.

- Find a short third eye meditation on YouTube to do every day.

- Visualize a tight rosebud at your forehead, and then in your mind's eye, visualize it opening and expanding.

- Ask open-ended questions and release the need to get a "profound" answer. Then just observe what comes into your thoughts. With yes-or-no questions you will have an attachment to the answer, so be sure to ask open-ended questions, such as "What do I need to know today?" or "What can I do to move myself forward?" Write down what you notice. It could be a color, a feeling, a chill, a smile, or a sentence. Don't judge or have preconceived notions about what sort of response you should get. Just observe and make it a daily practice to build that intuition "muscle."

Crown Chakra

The crown chakra represents your spiritual awareness—not a religious awareness necessarily, but more of a "Universe-y" awareness. It's our connection to Source/Spirit/God. The crown chakra is where our divine inspiration comes in, and is our connection to loved ones who have passed. If this area is closed, it can result in a feeling of hopelessness and victimization when it comes to getting pregnant. When deciding to try an alternative approach to fertility, you must be open to the idea that things could change, that you're supported by the Universe/God, and that by shifting your thoughts you can shift your circumstances. In order to manifest, we need to remember this connection. We are having a human experience, but we are still connected to Source. It can be helpful to be aware of that connection, as it can aid you in unexpected ways.

Here are some things you can do to open/strengthen your crown chakra:

- Visualize a white, gold, or purple light being poured in through your crown chakra from a pitcher above your head. Ask to let in the energy and information that is for your highest good and to receive whatever guidance you need.

- Ask for the help of your guides, angels, and/or loved ones who have passed for guidance or signs (without the attachment of needing to get an answer right away). Mantras can be helpful to open you up, break old thought patterns, and connect you to universal energy. Try something like this: "I invite in the next step," or "I am excited for Source/Spirit/God to unfold the next step in my journey," or "I am open to receiving the messages that help me move forward."

- Try automatic writing. Take a couple minutes to meditate and get your body still. Loosely hold a pen to paper and ask an open-ended question, like "What next step should I take?" or "What do I need to know today?" Again, you don't want to ask a yes-or-no question, because you'll be attached to one of those answers and that can skew the results. Don't judge what comes up; just write. It's okay if you don't get anything right away. It took me about three weeks of writing every day to get consistent messages. It's more about building the pattern of *allowing* in the message versus *hunting* for it. These are two very different energies, as we've already discussed. Automatic writing gets you in the habit of tapping into this amazing invisible team you have, who are just waiting for you to ask for and receive their help. If you're religious, tap into your angels. If you're spiritual, tap into your spirit guides. If you were close to a family member who passed, tap into that person.

It's so easy in this day and age to be caught up in external things, like work, relationships, and responsibilities, that we rarely make the time to listen to and energize ourselves. You can take action to move yourself forward in a positive way by listening to chakra meditations and simply visualizing the color of each chakra spinning, beginning at the root chakra and working up to the crown. This is something that can affect not only your fertility but every area of your life. Again, this journey is really about taking care of you and moving yourself forward. Going inward to replenish and recharge yourself will make what has seemed a daunting journey much more doable.

6

········

Case Studies

An in-depth glimpse into client victories

I'd like to share with you the case studies of seven of my clients who did some amazing work and were able to get pregnant. All of these women were dealing with elements of all four parts discussed so far in this book: (1) external factors, (2) beliefs, (3) physical conditions, and (4) Law of Attraction issues. All of these women have felt everything you've felt. And while something different "clicked" for each of them, it's important to read their stories and see that they had all but given up hope—but they made it happen. They were able to feel empowered with their new tools and step out and choose this. Their names have been changed for privacy's sake, but here are their journeys.

Before we begin, let me take a minute to say that I am not bashing IVF (in vitro fertilization). For some women, that's the right route. This book, though, is for women who want a less invasive approach. I have clients who want to do IVF but also work with me to increase their chances of conceiving. So whatever you want to do is great. These are stories of women who were told that IVF was their only option, and they conceived naturally anyway.

Gemma

Gemma's story is one we discussed in previous chapters. I had been working primarily with people with chronic pain and cancer at the time, and was actually supposed to do a session on her husband's faulty knees. He decided he wasn't really open to the idea, so I asked Gemma if she'd be interested in doing a session. In my work with clients with chronic pain, I work from the main principle that there's always an emotional cause to the physical problem, and that when that emotional issue is addressed, the physical condition no longer needs to be there. And I thought, "Well, the same principle should apply for infertility. Even if there's no obvious physical condition, she physically can't get pregnant, so there has to be something emotional going on."

Now, while I love Gemma, I didn't necessarily expect her to say yes to a session. I've been met with a lot of skepticism in my day, and I thought I'd be met with more of the same. But she happily agreed, so away we went.

She had been trying for two years to get pregnant; and she had in fact gotten pregnant twice, but those pregnancies had ended in miscarriage at seven and eleven weeks. She was scared she'd never get pregnant again, but she was also scared to *be* pregnant after the trauma of the other two losses.

As we began the energy work portion, I could feel her relax, but I honestly wasn't sure what she'd get from it—if she could let herself go in the process. But I kept working and noted the intuitive hits that I was getting. Then it came time for the notes portion of the session where I go over the information I got, where it resonates for the client, and how we move forward. I didn't know if she was going to be able to hear what came up or if she'd get defensive or shut down, etc. But before I could speak she said, "I saw purple-blue light at my forehead and orange light at my lower abdomen." She knew nothing about chakras, yet those happen to be the colors for those exact energy centers. She also felt warmth and some involuntary twitching (twitching is the energy that was stuck kicking through—always a good sign!). I felt encouraged that she had gotten so many feelings and visuals out of the first session, so I felt more empowered giving her the notes, trusting that she would hear whatever she was supposed to hear.

I won't go into what came up at each chakra, but it's important to note that four of the areas fit into the four categories discussed in this book: external factors, beliefs, physical conditions, and Law of Attraction issues.

External Factors

At the solar plexus chakra, which is the power center (in my experience, this usually has to do with work), I was seeing Gemma at her school teaching. But the important thing about the visual was that she had eight arms. Yeah, eight. One was writing on the chalkboard, one was passing out papers, one extended into her office for a department head meeting, one was holding the summer school schedule, etc. So it was pretty clear to me that she was over-extended at work. She had her fingers in too many pies. I asked her where this made sense for her, and she confirmed that she had the following things going on: teacher at an inner-city high school, department head, teaching two extra AP classes, teaching summer school, taking two graduate classes, and teaching a continuing education class at a local college.

Whew! That's a lot. So I asked her, where was the room for the baby in all of this? She said, "Well obviously I'd change it if I were pregnant." I lovingly pointed out that it was a major factor why she wasn't getting pregnant. When your brain/ego already feels like there isn't enough time and you're stretched too thin, your survival mechanism kicks in and it thinks it's doing you a favor by not allowing in yet another thing to take care of. I told Gemma, "Fix it now. Make an energetic change now. Even if you can't quit everything right now, there are adjustments you can make."

So Gemma made some changes. She weaned herself off some of her obligations and showed the Universe that she was making room for this baby.

Beliefs

Gemma had a bunch of beliefs come up, as many of us do, but her two main beliefs were "I'm going to be an old mom/I'm running out of time" and "I'm going to have another miscarriage because the last two were."

Beliefs are tricky little buggers because while they are just thoughts, the brain accepts them as true. Society has told us that thirty-five years old is too late to have a baby and that our pregnancy will be fraught with danger. While there are cases of things going wrong, that's the exception, not the rule. And frankly there are other factors involved besides age when special circumstances arise. Despite it being plausible for a woman in Europe to have a healthy birth at age fifty, in the US it's somewhat taboo. And we've been plugging into that belief for a long time. It's very likely that our parents, friends, and family all buy into this belief.

So for Gemma, she was worried about complications and didn't want to be judged for being an old, not hip, can't-keep-up type of mom. In reality, she's a fashion-forward, energetic go-getter. So once we did some belief work, she was able to let go of these ideas.

Physical Conditions

Gemma had also dealt with a number of physical issues, including two miscarriages, thyroid issues, dangerously thin uterine lining, residual scar tissue from miscarriages, and an inability to get more than three follicles when attempting IUI. Let's look at them one at a time.

Miscarriage, as I've mentioned, has to do with not being ready or the timing not being right. Gemma was so ready to be a mom that how could she not be ready, right? Well, here's an example of where plugging into beliefs can cause physical issues. Gemma is a teacher, and one of the women she worked with was talking about having kids and said, "Oh I had two miscarriages before I could have a child." Gemma later said that she subconsciously knew at that moment that that's what would happen to her. The fear kicked in and she called that exact scenario into her experience.

It was after this that the thyroid issue popped up. Thyroid issues have to do with humiliation and feeling like "When's it going to be my turn?" Gemma has two master's degrees and is by all accounts an overachiever. She's used to being good at pretty much everything she does. But she wasn't "good" at being pregnant, so then the thyroid condition developed.

After trying several rounds of IUI, she was told she had residual scar tissue from her previous D&Cs. They told her she'd have to have another procedure to remove that before they could proceed with another IUI. We worked on some visualizations and mantras, and she was able to pass the scar tissue in her next cycle. This is when I really knew she was going to get pregnant, because if she could will herself to do that, she could do the same for a baby.

Then the doctors told her that her uterine lining was dangerously thin. They recommended she take soy, which she did; but as I mentioned before, too much soy isn't good. So again, she did some visualizations and positive thinking and her uterine lining doubled.

At the next IUI, she had three follicles and was all excited. That is until the tech came in and said, "Whew, the woman before you had eighteen, but you have … three! That's great." Gemma immediately felt like a failure, and because she couldn't help plugging into the thought-less words of the tech, that IUI cycle was never going to work. So we did some more deep-diving sessions and found that her brain was really scared to be pregnant. She had "failed" twice, something had been very wrong with the second pregnancy, and she'd had two scary surgeries. Her brain was in self-preservation mode. It wanted to keep her alive, and the safest way to do that (according to the brain) was to not be pregnant. It became very clear in my reading, however, that miscarriage wouldn't happen again. When she got pregnant this time, it would work. I then got a beautiful visual of her two miscarried ones as toddlers in a garden. They were a boy and a girl, and they were happy and smiling. In between them was a little baby, and they were swinging her back and forth, saying, "Whenever you're ready, Mom." This really landed emotionally for Gemma. It really struck a chord and something shifted. At her next IUI, guess how many follicles she had? Eighteen. The exact number the other woman had the last time.

Law of Attraction Issues

But there was something still blocking Gemma. She began to get frustrated and was looking into IVF. Her husband's insurance didn't cover IVF, so there was a wait period while she switched over to her insurance. During this time we had some more sessions and dug into where she was putting her energy. As humans it's so easy to focus on what's going wrong versus what's going right, and Gemma was no different. She was focusing on how awful work was, that it was hard to get pregnant, that she should have been pregnant by now, and that it was never going to happen. And listen, it's understandable when something you really want seems like it will never be in reach. So we began talking about the Law of Attraction and how the Universe responds with situations and experiences that are a direct match to what you're putting out. If you're not getting the results you want, it's time to look at where you're putting your energy.

One of the visuals that came up for her in our energy work was that she was outside on a beautiful day and she had a parka, snowshoes, an umbrella, galoshes, and pretty much everything you can imagine you'd need in inclement weather. But it was a gorgeous day, with no bad weather in sight, and yet she was preparing for the worst, saying over and over "Please don't rain, please don't snow." As we discussed earlier, the Universe doesn't hear the "don't" in "don't want." It hears what you're focusing on, in this case the rain and snow. So it started raining and snowing in this visual. It was matching her focus. Once she began to understand that and start redirecting her thoughts to things like "I've beaten all these other physical conditions, so I can do this as well," "I have a normal cycle," "I'm capable," and "I deserve to have the things I want in life," she was able to pull out of the wheel-spinning energy that was driving her crazy.

Then one gorgeous spring night we were at an outdoor wedding and Gemma asked me to come sit by the bonfire with her. As she gazed into the fire, she very matter-of-factly asked me if there are some people/ instances where it's just not biologically possible to get pregnant. I just as matter-of-factly answered, "No." She looked at me with a mix of surprise and hope. As discussed throughout the book, every physical issue is the result of an emotional block, and once that block is removed, the physical condition doesn't need to be there anymore. Can everyone do this? Technically, yes. If you have at least one ovary and a uterus, you can do this. *Will* everyone? No. A lot of people are not aware enough to get out of their own way—to step back from the fearsome thought, look at "what is," and decide to lean toward what they want. It's a foreign concept to most people, but if you shift your thought process, you can shift your physical condition. She looked at me and then into the fire and said, "Huh." *That night* is the night she got pregnant. Clearly something in that talk registered for her, and she let go of some fear/blocks and allowed the baby in. The timing couldn't have been more perfect, as she was about to go in for IVF the following month. She managed to figure it out in that little window of time and conceived naturally.

After Gemma told the people closest her the news and was done bouncing around excitedly, the old fears start to creep in: "The last two didn't work. What if this one doesn't?" Every little pang, twinge, and cramp was scary to her, and how could it not be considering what she'd been through? That's when the spotting began. During her previous pregnancies, spotting had begun at six and eleven weeks. At the start of week seven, I got a panicked phone call from her at work saying, "It's happening again!"

Here's where the belief work and the Law of Attraction were absolutely key. She was focusing on not wanting spotting—but she was looking for spotting, so the Universe heard "I'm looking for spotting" and had to answer with what was being requested. So we focused on her victories: that she had released scar tissue, doubled her uterine lining, tripled the number of follicles, and healed her thyroid condition—which reminded her that *she* was in control of her body. If she thought scary things and something "bad" started to happen, then she could think good thoughts and "good" things would happen. We talked about how she was in a different place this time and why the other pregnancies hadn't worked out but this one would.

Then we did a form of the belief work. I asked her who would she be/what would she think if she couldn't think the thought "It's happening again." It took her a minute to calm her breath and step outside of her current fear. Then she said, "Well, spotting is a normal part of the first trimester. It's not weird or unusual to have spotting at the beginning." When I asked her how she'd feel if that were the case, I felt her energy melt as she said, "Relieved. Like I'm gonna be okay. Excited. Still riding off the high of what I just achieved by getting pregnant!" Abso-freakin-lutely! I asked her which way would get her what she wanted, thinking that it's happening again or not thinking that? She replied, "Not thinking it. If I'm thinking it, I'm reaping what I sow. Law of Attraction—wise, I'm attracting that no matter what. If I decide it's normal, there's at least a chance it'll be fine." Exactly right. It's not delusional or wishful thinking if you feel into what's going right, the relief, and then knowing that everything is fine. You have zero chance the other way, so why not lean toward what feels good?

Then we moved on to the turnaround work. If the belief is *It's (miscarrying) happening again*, then the turnaround is *It's NOT happening again*.

I had her give me three reasons why it could hypothetically be true that it wasn't happening again. Here's what she came up with:

- I've done a lot of work on myself and am in a different mental space than I was before. I know I'm ready now.

- The spotting isn't heavy and spotting is normal in the first trimester.

- I'm deciding that it's not happening. If we choose everything that comes in, then I am choosing that everything is fine. When I close my eyes and connect to this baby, I know she's fine. I chose to move through all the other physical things and didn't conquer all that to not go all the way.

Suddenly Gemma was empowered in what up until a few minutes earlier was the worst situation she could have imagined, and *by the end of the school day, the spotting had stopped.* Let me be clear that if Gemma hadn't pulled herself out of this spiral by calling me and being willing to do the work to shift her energy, she would have stayed in "It's happening again," and she would very likely have had her third miscarriage. This is especially important for those of you who have had multiple miscarriages. It's admittedly scary to realize you have control over the situation, but I hope you can see how empowering it can be. When you realize that it's not some "thing in the sky" or punishment or karma keeping this baby from you, but that by shifting your thoughts you can shift your physical condition via the Law of Psychophysical Response, you can decide that this thing you want is happening. That is so freaking exciting to me, and it's the most amazing thing when my clients have that aha moment. Gemma is the poster child for this work as far as I'm concerned. She went on to apply these techniques to all areas of her life and is now a chill mom with an amazing baby, and she loves life right now. She made that choice. And you can do it too.

Jenny

After Jenny saw an article I wrote for MindBodyGreen, she sent me an email that started with "I was about to give up until I read your article this morning." There was something about Jenny from the start where I knew I had to work with her. Like Gemma, she was dealing with a combination of all four parts mentioned in this book: external factors, beliefs, physical conditions, and Law of Attraction issues.

External Factors

Jenny worked for her father's business and so did her husband. There was a lot of stress for her being a mediator between her father and husband. She felt caught in the middle, like she couldn't speak up. She didn't like how she and her husband were being treated but didn't know how to get out of it. After all, it was the family business. She loved her dad, but was really feeling like this wasn't the right place for her anymore.

When I asked her "If money didn't matter right now and you could be whatever you wanted, what would you do?" Jenny answered with such passion that she wanted to be a holistic health coach and had just completed her training. Her husband was supportive, but she didn't have enough confidence in herself that she could make it a viable business, enough to leave her dad's business. So we did some belief work around that for her to be able to at least entertain the idea that this was possible, and then began building her business little by little.

Jenny was also completely overscheduling herself. She'd wake up super-early to work out, train clients, write programs for them, go to work for eight hours, come home, make dinner, do laundry, clean up, and then go to bed. To her brain, there was no breathing room there. She was just trying to stay afloat, so how on earth could she add a child to the mix? Where would the baby fit in? How would they take care of her? So her brain said, "Since you're overscheduled as it is, let's not add anything else to the mix."

So we had to look at her schedule and see where we could make space. Laundry and cleaning were both relegated to one day per week. With some difficulty she resisted the urge to clean and straighten up in the evenings so she could spend time with the hubby watching a movie, etc. We had to carve out some respite time so her body wasn't constantly in a state of stress or "go mode." It was energetically important to make space for the baby.

Beliefs

Oh boy, Jenny had a lot of them—as we all do, really. Perhaps you can relate to some of these:

- I'm not going to be able to have my own child.

- It should have happened by now.

- If it were going to happen, it would have by now.

- I've mistreated my body, so it's not capable anymore.

- This next IUI *has* to work.

Here is some work she did with the belief that she should have been pregnant by now (using a belief sheet).

Belief: *I should be pregnant by now.*

Is it true? Yes.

Can you be 1,000 percent sure that you're probably going to get your period this month (feel into it)? No.

How do you feel when you think that thought? (Close your eyes and notice your muscles, breathing, and where that feeling shows up in your body.): Heavy pressure and tightness in my chest, hollow in my lower abdomen. Nervous, panicky, running out of time. Not fair. Like a failure, incomplete.

How do you show up/who are you being in your life when you think that thought? How does it affect your life when you think that thought? Stuck. Can't move forward because I'm so stuck in the past with what I think should have happened. Resigned because I feel like I've missed my window. Pissed because why is everyone else good enough to get pregnant and I can't? Shut down. What's the point?

Who/How would you be if you COULDN'T think that thought? How would you FEEL in your body and show up in life? If I couldn't think that I was probably going to get it? I'd feel lighter in my chest—like a flutter of excitement that it must be coming soon. I'd feel ready to offload the baggage that's holding me back because I know it's gonna move me forward that much faster. I'd just be feeling into all those good, squishy feelings that she's coming and I can't wait.

Which way is going to get you what you want: thinking the thought that you should have been pregnant by now or not thinking the thought? Why? Not thinking the thought. Because then I'm focused on the thing I don't want. I'm focusing on the negative. And if I'm feeling negative about the situation, I'm attracting negative *to* the situation.

The turnaround. Can you find three examples of where the opposite of your belief is true? (Ex. If the belief is "My boyfriend makes me mad," the turnarounds are "I make my boyfriend mad. My boyfriend makes me happy. I make *me* mad.") I shouldn't be pregnant by now. I'll be pregnant soon when the timing is right. My thinking should be pregnant by now.

Can you find three examples where each turnaround is/could be true?

I shouldn't be pregnant by now.

- I shouldn't be pregnant by now because I'm not. If I should be pregnant by now, I would be. I'm not, so there's something else for me to do or learn first. It doesn't mean it won't happen, but it hasn't been the right time up until now.

- I've overworked and mistreated my body for years, and while I've been better, I need to give it more recovery time. (Jenny was a bodybuilder and had dealt with disordered eating for many years, which we will discuss in the next section).

- I'm just now getting the courage to build my own business and voice what I need from my job and family. If I were pregnant by now, I probably wouldn't have had the courage to do all those things that are going to benefit me as a person and as a mother.

I'll be pregnant soon when the timing is right.

- As I already mentioned, I am getting my new business, which is my passion, in place. It will allow me more freedom and flexibility in my schedule, which will benefit my baby.

- Even though my reflex is to want to control everything, I can't possibly know what my timeline is. All I can do is be open to the things that come down the pipes, knowing that they're leading me to my baby.

- I'm doing all of this mindfulness work and shifting my energy, so I will be pregnant soon because I'm taking positive steps to move myself forward toward what I want. And if I'm focusing on definitely being pregnant when the timing is right, the Universe has to respond with those circumstances, right?

My thinking should be pregnant by now.

- My brain thinks that I have too much going on and that if it were possible, it would have happened already. But that's the fight-or-flight getting triggered.

- My ego—my control—thinks it should have happened. And the more I give in to that, the more miserable I am. So I need to start filling my intuition with pregnant thoughts.

- My friends are all getting pregnant and having babies now, and I guess my brain thinks I should be there as well. So when I don't plug into that, it's not stressful and I can just be on my own timeline.

Whenever the belief you're working with starts with "I," most of the time you can replace "I" with "My thinking." This is a good way to make it less about you failing and more about separating your ego/brain from your intuition. It helps delineate that it's not your being that's misaligned, it's just your thoughts—your thinking. Having this type of turnaround makes it easier to step back and address the belief from a less personal, less "blamey," more exploratory way. This type of turnaround was really useful for Jenny, and she focused on the phrase "I am not my thoughts." It's so true. We have plugged into programming from society, our parents, and our past experiences. So to have a tool like this to separate herself from the "yuck" was really helpful for Jenny.

Physical Conditions

As already mentioned, Jenny had dealt with disordered eating for many years and was a bodybuilder. So her body had been pushed to the limit for years on end, and this had caused various physical things to happen in her body that were not conducive to conception.

She had amenorrhea, which, as discussed in chapter 3, is the absence of blood. So she was not getting a cycle on her own, even after conquering the eating disorder and toning down her workouts. In Jenny's case, the emotional cause of her amenorrhea was denying her femininity in a masculine field, both with bodybuilding and work. The eating disorder contributed heavily to this, and often occurs when we feel like we don't have control in one or more areas of our life, so what can we control?

Every single thing that goes in our body. While Jenny had utter control over her body when she felt out of control elsewhere, through breakups and other life changes, her body had been pushed to the limit in terms of survival. Having a child was the last thing her brain thought she could handle, so why have a period?

Related to this was a low-functioning hypothalamus gland. The hypothalamus, as I mentioned, is the control center and links the nervous system to the endocrine system via the pituitary gland. If these are not functioning at proper levels, the areas that they govern—like the adrenals (fight-or-flight), the thyroid, and the ovaries—will not perform normally. This is what was happening with Jenny. So we did some work on her need to control things and how that was physically affecting her. I also had her apply Clary Sage oil by Young Living every day to the place where her head meets her neck and on her lower abdomen. Within one month she was having a cycle on her own—unmedicated. That hadn't happened in over seven years. It was then, I think, that she really thought there was a chance of conceiving naturally.

Jenny also led the charge on backing off on the frequency and intensity of her workouts to let her body rest and gain some fat that she would need to have a healthy baby. She started doing that on her own because she was ready. She wanted the baby now more than she wanted the perfect body, and she put her fears aside and went into feminine/nurture mode.

Another physical condition that was an issue involved Jenny's husband. He was dealing with low sperm count and motility. You already learned about the various causes of this condition in chapter 3. In his case, it was being unhappy in his job. As I mentioned, it's hard to work with family sometimes and he was feeling caught between a rock and a hard place. Plus his real dream was to be a firefighter, but the county they lived in wasn't hiring. So I suggested he look into volunteer brigades and to start feeling into how awesome it was going to be when he was doing what he loves to do for a career. Sometimes when we're so mired down in what we don't like, we forget to put energy toward our dreams. Frustration inhibits creation, and his ability to create a human was diminished because of his frustration around providing. He was also a trooper and used the Idaho Blue Spruce oil by Young Living at night so as not to "smell like a hippie" (wink). Sometimes husbands are not so open to alternative methods, but he was willing to do whatever was necessary.

Both Jenny and her husband had encountered their share of insensitive doctors who had diminished their chances and ruined their mood at every turn, exacerbating the situation. So they finally changed doctors and she started seeing a midwife. All of a sudden her hormones had regulated, and his morphology wasn't so concerning. It seems they were both plugging into the doom and gloom presented by the previous care providers.

Law of Attraction Issues

Each time Jenny would go in for clomid or an IUI, she would go in with the energy of "This *has* to work." Now, that may sound like a positive pep talk, but it's actually the opposite. According to the Law of Attraction, whatever energy you're putting out there, the Universe has to respond to with like energy. "This *has* to be it" means "I'm really worried that it's not going to be it, and I'm desperate for it to be it." And *that's* what the Universe hears—the desperation, fear, and longing—not what you *say*. So each IUI would fail because she was calling in that wonky energy. It's a subtlety that's tricky to catch but super-important to understand.

Once we did some work on those subtleties and she felt more in control of her process when she accepted that her results were directly related to her energy (and not in a blaming way), she began to get stronger and more positive and not go in with the attachment to it working but rather the feeling that wouldn't it be awesome if it did?

Then one of her doctors said that with her husband's sperm motility, IVF was really going to be her only option. We were all disappointed, but she decided to do it. However, we kept working on her energy, as IVF is not a guarantee, and we wanted to help make the procedure as viable as possible. So for the month before her first IVF blood work appointment, we focused on putting out the energy that she was nourishing her body, was healthy, was going to make an amazing mom, etc.

Then the day came for Jenny to go in for her blood work. The nurse came back to her and said, "Um, you're pregnant. About four weeks, I'd say." Whoa! How amazing is that! Just like with Gemma, during that little window of time before the procedure, something clicked for Jenny and she made it happen. I was over the moon when she called me and I screamed at the top of my lungs in the middle of the Cheesecake Factory. It was so exciting and so amazing to see that by changing your thoughts and the way you're putting your energy out there, you can overcome years of physical damage and anxiety, even when your partner is part of the "infertility" factor.

Jenny continued to have some scary thoughts and anxiety throughout the first trimester, but all it took was a session or a quick text or email to get her back on track. What really got her through was reminding her to listen to her body, that she was not her scary thoughts, and to put out the energy that she wanted back. She embraced her pregnant body and had a beautiful pregnancy. Jenny gave birth to a beautiful baby boy, and a year and a half later gave birth to baby number two! She chose the pregnancy over the fear. And you can too, mama.

Chloe

Chloe was actually in one of my music classes in high school. After not seeing each other for seventeen years and living on opposite ends of the country, she saw one of my Facebook posts about my work and sent me an email.

She had been "trying" (we need to come up with a better word) for over a year and was starting to get really disheartened. She had done one IUI that didn't work, and doctors told her IVF was her only option. She refused to believe that, and reached out to me.

It may not be a surprise at this point, but Chloe was also dealing with a combination of the four parts discussed in this book: external factors, beliefs, physical conditions, and Law of Attraction issues.

External Factors

Chloe taught music, English, and theater at a high school. She had a lot going on besides the standard workweek; there were concerts, play rehearsals, etc. She had zero time for anything else and was feeling burned-out. As often happens with teachers who are super-involved, the brain thinks, "We have no time for anything else, so how are we going to manage a baby? Plus you already have fifty kids! Why are we adding another thing to your plate?" It's no wonder she wasn't getting pregnant, with tons of stress and no time to herself.

So she decided to quit that job and teach music lessons from home. While that was less stressful in multiple respects, if you've ever owned your own business, you know that a lot of work goes into getting it off the ground and you need to take care of it like a baby. So her brain thought, "You already have a baby, so why do we need to make another one?"

To help Chloe stop running around like a chicken with its head cut off, we worked on techniques to drop her back into her body and begin to listen to her intuition more. She considers herself an intuitive person, but sometimes when issues like fertility are a little too close to you, that can go out the window. I had her get some specific stones and write her baby a song to really connect to the baby's energy and plug into knowing she could do this versus worrying about what if she couldn't.

Beliefs

It was hard for Chloe not to plug into the percentages—of fertility, of interventions, of risk. It's especially hard when doctors, society, and family (though well-meaning) remind us continually that it's unlikely we'll be successful. When she heard that IUI had an 18 percent success rate, she realized that she never really thought it would work because her brain decided the chances were so slim, what was the point of getting excited about it?

She was also dealing with the common belief that she "should be pregnant by now." A lot of her energy was going toward something that she thought should have already happened, but the fact was, it hadn't happened, so it shouldn't have. Once we looked at why that might be true (having a stressful job, quitting that and starting her own business, moving, etc.), she was able to let go of that energy and move forward. Anything that stresses us out isn't true, so when we can step back and look at why it was perfect and purposeful the way it happened, we are able to move forward much faster.

Physical Conditions

Though Chloe had no physical issues, her husband was dealing with low sperm count and motility. Unlike Jenny's husband, he was not comfortable trying alternative methods, so we had to use a less direct approach with him (so not to worry if your partner is similar to Chloe's!). Honestly most of this work is energetically about you anyway, but here's what we did for Chloe's husband.

She started giving her husband massages with Mister essential oil by Young Living, which can help regulate his hormones. Unbeknownst to him, he was receiving the benefits. She put two stones specifically for his issues (ruby-in-zoisite and black coral) under his mattress. Luckily he wasn't like the princess in *The Princess and the Pea*, and he didn't feel them! And while cuddling him at night, she'd put a hand on his heart and energetically encourage him to release whatever wasn't serving him anymore. In a subsequent reading, it came up that he was drinking too much beer. He wasn't an alcoholic by any means, but too much beer can decimate the sperm count. So Chloe broached the subject with him about quitting alcohol for a couple of months, and *poof!* She went in for her next IUI and she was pregnant! Once she was no longer hung up about the percentages, she allowed herself to be open to the procedure actually working.

Law of Attraction Issues

Chloe got caught up in the energy of "I'm probably never going to be a mother." Between what her doctors had told her and what her experience had been, she was quickly losing hope, and that energy was gaining momentum fast. So part of our work was clearing her energy with reiki and then using mindset coaching to move her through the beliefs that were attracting more and more of this resigned, give-up kind of energy. She realized that there were a lot of reasons why she *would* get pregnant and began to align her energy with the excitement of finding out that she was pregnant by starting a private wish list on Babies R Us and Baby Earth to get into the energy that this baby was coming. We're taught not to count our chickens before they hatch, but that's exactly what you want to do, as long as you stay in the energy of knowing that they'll hatch versus hoping they will. Hoping is scared and not in control. Your energy needs to be in a place of "I've decided this is happening. I deserve it, and I invite the next step in."

Her energy also took a bit of a dip when she found out that her husband had male factor infertility. She understandably felt helpless and at a loss because she knew he wasn't open to alternative methods and she really didn't want to put herself through IVF. Chloe's energy began to spiral until we discussed the subtle methods to help her help her husband that we just mentioned. And the more positive and open her energy was, the more her husband's energy followed suit. She could have just been upset and wallowed in how unfair the situation was, but she aligned herself with what she wanted versus what she didn't want. It was no longer a matter of *if* she got pregnant but *when*.

Chloe didn't expect an easy fix. She did the work and committed to strengthening her intuition and aligning herself with the solution instead of the problem. It takes a long time for this to become second nature, but it's the only way to pull out of the helpless, wheel-spinning energy.

Chloe gave birth to a beautiful baby girl and, looking back, is so glad she quit a stressful job and took the time to build a business that she loves, and that everything was in place when the baby got here. It helped her feel stable, solid, and capable, and when you ask her about it now, she says she wouldn't have wanted the journey to be any other way.

Amy

Amy was in what doctors would call the unexplained fertility group. My clients who fall into this group often say they almost wish they had something physical because then at least they'd know what they were dealing with. It's frustrating for nothing medical or physical to show up as wrong but still have difficulty getting pregnant.

Part of my job is to get in there and find out what emotional blocks are inhibiting the process. What are the external factors, beliefs, and Law of Attraction issues in play that we are just not able to consciously see in ourselves? When our issues are so deep-rooted, it's not always obvious what they are, where they come from, and what we should do about them.

Here's what came up when working with Amy and how she moved through her blocks.

External Factors

In the three years since Amy and her husband got married, they had been working on starting a family. She couldn't understand why it wasn't happening. In one of my initial sessions with her, it came up that her solar plexus chakra was closed.

The solar plexus is the power center and is connected to drive and ambition. When I'm reading people, it usually represents work/career, so to me, finding this area closed means there's something going on at work. It turns out that Amy and her husband had both changed jobs and moved to a new house around the same time, and she found herself working as a dental hygienist in a very toxic work environment, which was kicking up her anxiety big time. As I've mentioned, when your fight-or-flight response is constantly turned on, the *last* thing your brain wants to do is add a baby to the mix. Again, it's trying to do you a favor by not creating more stress, so it sends messages to the endocrine and nervous systems to slow down, and that's what was happening for her.

We also took a look at whether she was in the career she wanted to be in or in one she felt obligated to be in. Amy answered pretty quickly that it was her dream to be a yoga instructor. That's quite a shift from a dental office, and she wasn't sure how to go about it or if she should go for it. Well, she found a certification class, but she got pregnant after our very first session, so the certification had to wait. But just knowing that she would eventually pursue her purpose versus remaining in a job she felt obligated to do was very freeing energetically, and clearly helped move things forward.

Beliefs

It took me a few sessions to really tune in and dig deep to figure out that most of the beliefs Amy was carrying around were not actually hers, but her mother's. Again, when it comes to parents, we want to keep in mind that they did the best they could with the skills and limitations they had. But from as far back as Amy can remember, her mother was very strict, fearful, and controlling. Everything Amy did was controlled by her mother, so Amy grew up very fearful and distrusting of life, convinced that something was constantly out to get her or that something bad would happen if she strayed too far from home. This developed into almost debilitating anxiety. When anxiety is kicked up, the fight-or-flight reflex is active, so the body slows or shuts down all unnecessary processes in the body. Remember, the brain's main concern is keeping you alive. And when you're in a state of constant panic, the last thing your brain thinks you need is to be adding another responsibility to your life. So on top of Amy's already present anxiety, she was having anxiety about not being able to get pregnant.

The great thing about this belief/mindset work is that it really helps you step back and look at what is, versus the doomsday, apocalyptic fears our brain manufactures. The fears our brain creates to "keep us safe" are often way scarier than what actually *is*. And once we realize that we are okay and that the things that are freaking us out aren't actually true, our body is able to come out of flight-or-flight mode and feel safe enough to make a baby.

So with this work we were able to deconstruct these beliefs enough for Amy to get pregnant. It was super-exciting! Not only was she pregnant, but she had much less anxiety about going out and experiencing life.

And then … she found out she was having twins. That kicked up her anxiety big time. So we did some more work and it turned out that her mother had told Amy that she'd probably have to be on bed rest, and her doctor had said it was very likely that one twin would take nutrients from the other, so she should plan to deliver early and would probably have to have a C-section because it's hard to deliver twins naturally. Well, jeez! Even though there was no ill intent on the part of the doctor, this is yet another example of how medical personnel can exacerbate the situation by not being aware of how they phrase things. Amy's head was spinning and she immediately defaulted to the idea that her body wasn't capable.

And this is where a lot of women get stuck: they default to the beliefs of family or doctors and don't listen to their own body. It's not their fault; we're trained that way. But believing those things to be true was causing stress in Amy's body and was going to cause those exact things to manifest.

So we looked at the fact that Amy was in great physical shape and there was no physical reason she would have to deliver early. Twins can easily go to thirty-seven weeks, which is considered full term, and she was not going to make babies that she couldn't deliver. While tuning in to her body, I picked up pretty early on that the babies were boys and that one of them was kind of a show-off and a smart-ass and the other was a little more straight-laced and calm. This made it easier for her to do visualizations to talk to them, which kept her calm and already in mom mode. It became about sending them love and getting them here safe, and she couldn't be in that place *and* a place of fear at the same time, so she was able to let go of the fear. I told her, "Way to manifest! You were shooting for one and you got two. That's pretty badass!" Soon after, she became excited about having twins (and they were both boys, by the way!).

It's hard not to plug into what family members and doctors say. A lot of times we don't even realize we've done it. And that is why this work is so important. It's a way to unearth, identify, and move through these beliefs (which aren't true) so you can conceive and have a peaceful pregnancy and birth.

The thing to keep in mind is that the things that family and doctors get freaked out about are the *exceptions*, not the *rule*. We can end up in that exception category if we believe these things will go wrong. Getting quiet with yourself and dropping into your body will help you know what's true and not a belief. This is an essential tool for moving forward. And I'm so proud of Amy for doing the work and having the natural birth they said wouldn't happen to twins who were the same size and healthy.

Physical Conditions

For many years Amy had dealt with an eating disorder. This isn't a surprise. Her mother had tried to control everything in her life, so the only thing Amy could control was what went into her body. Then the problem came back when her anxiety picked up. In a world that seemed out of control and where something bad could happen at any second, at least she could control what was going on with her body.

Identifying that correlation was very important for Amy. Even though she had healed quite a bit, the tendency would still be there if things got stressful. Luckily there were only a couple of relapses, and she was getting to the point where she was sick of having to be afraid, sick of monitoring it, and she wanted to get to what the actual root of the problem was.

On top of the fear of relapsing into the eating disorder, Amy was having strong physical reactions to her anxiety, to the point of having to go to the emergency room. But the doctors couldn't find anything wrong. These physical symptoms only amplified her anxiety that something was wrong, so we did some more work, and I tuned in to her body to see where there might be some physical issues. Nothing showed up. It was very clear to me that she was experiencing the Law of Psychophysical Response—where every thought has a corresponding physical reaction.

We talked about herbs, Bach Flower remedies, exercises, and visualizations that she could do on her own, in addition to the energy work and belief work we were doing in our sessions.

When you're that afraid, it's hard to step back and trust that things are going to be okay and that you are in control of your life. When it's an ingrained pattern, you might not be able to crack it right away or win every time at the beginning. But the more you practice leaning toward relief, toward what feels good, toward what you want versus what you don't, you'll go for longer and longer periods where you feel good and the anxiety isn't winning. It's taken Amy a few tries, but she gets better and better each time and is reclaiming control of her life.

Law of Attraction Issues

As I've mentioned, Amy was dealing with some pretty deep-rooted anxiety. The emotional cause of anxiety is not trusting the process of life and assuming things will go horribly wrong. This is more than being a glass-is-half-empty kind of person; this can seriously affect multiple areas of your life, including fertility.

Amy's anxiety was almost debilitating, and she had no idea why. Yes, she had changed jobs and moved and wasn't getting pregnant, but none of that was the cause of this paralyzing fear. Her friendships had been affected because she was afraid to go out, because "What if something happens? What if I have a panic attack and I'm too far from home? What if I have to go to the hospital?" The only way she would go out was if her husband gently forced her to socialize. He was very supportive but didn't know where this unjustified fear was coming from.

Amy told me that she knew they were unfounded fears, but they were so debilitating, and she couldn't help but think the worst would happen at every turn. What you've hopefully learned by now in this book is that whatever energy we are putting out into the Universe, we are getting back. So she was continually putting out that there was something to be afraid of, and the Universe answered with more fear and more things to be afraid of. In addition to her fear of an emergency happening, Amy was afraid her body would fail and something serious or life-threatening would happen to her. The energy Amy was putting out that "my body could fail me" returned to her with an example of her body "failing her" by not being able to get pregnant.

So we really had to work on retraining her brain and her energy to focus not on the problem but on the solution. And that's hard when it's an ingrained pattern that you've had for years. But that's why you might need someone like me to help you identify and move through it, because oftentimes we just can't see when we're falling into that negative spiral.

A simple shift from "What if something goes wrong?" to "What if something goes right?" makes all the difference in the world. Feel into what it would feel like if everything was, in fact, right and okay. That feeling of relief stops the spinning and makes it easier for us to move forward.

Once Amy realized that she was creating all of the experiences in her life, good, "bad," or otherwise, she felt more confident that she could step up to the plate and actually change her life. And she did.

Anna

Anna called me for the first time in tears. She had just been to a fertility specialist and was overwhelmed. They had told her she needed to get in for IVF immediately and that even that probably wouldn't work because of her age. Let's look at what was going on with Anna.

External Factors

Anna is from another country and is in the US on a visa. She is not in a profession she likes anymore. In fact, she never liked it—it was what her parents wanted her to do. This job wasn't filling her soul, but she didn't know what else to do, as she needed to stay in the country a certain amount of time to get her citizenship. So we began to look at things she could do to fulfill herself and also to set her energy toward something that would really light her up. She also wasn't living in a place that was conducive to having children, and her fiancé lived in their home country, so she was feeling unsafe and her fight-or-flight response was triggered.

Beliefs

Having a narcissistic mother was difficult for Anna, especially being an empath who feels everything. There were some beliefs about her worth and capability that came up, as well as processing what the doctors had just smacked her in the face with. As long as she believed these things, her situation would stay the same, so we had to shift them through the belief work. Thoughts like "I'm running out of time," "I have to stay in my current job, which I don't like," and "I won't be able to do this without IVF" would have consumed her and kept her stuck. But by examining, dismantling, and turning around these thoughts, she was able to move forward.

Physical Conditions

Anna was very healthy. She ate well, exercised, and took care of herself. However, she was forty years old, and the doctors were extremely concerned and wanted to hurry because they assumed her egg count would be diminished (without even looking, by the way).

Law of Attraction Issues

When we met, Anna was very much in a place of fear. She wanted to give her fiancé a child and had basically been told it was impossible, and certainly not without IVF. Naturally, Anna started to believe this might be true, and she was devastated. Remember that it's only the thoughts about the situation that are scary, not what actually *is*. When she was caught up in the thought that it was over for her, it was unbearable. When she stepped back and looked at what was going *right,* she was able to say, "I have a normal cycle. I'm healthy. My fiancé loves me and I can't wait to see him next month. Deep down I know my body was made for this, and I can do this." It can be hard to go to that positive place when you're stressed-out, but you must in order to shift the energy. Even if you can hold the positive thought for only thirty seconds one day, that's something! Maybe the next day it will be two minutes, then twenty minutes, and then an hour. From a Law of Attraction perspective, if like energy attracts like energy, then focusing on what's going right brings more things going right. Focusing on what's going wrong brings more things going wrong.

So Anna worked on this for a month and then took a trip home to see her fiancé. She pretty much got pregnant the second she could! She was so excited when she came back to the US—and then it happened. She was back at her job, which she hated, and in a living situation that wasn't good, not to mention she was without her fiancé. She began to miscarry. It was, of course, heartbreaking, but those conditions we mentioned needed to be addressed, and she knew it.

Despite her pain and disappointment, Anna knew that on a deeper level this was happening for a reason. We discussed making some big moves at work that seemed risky to everyone else but felt true for her. She went back home and was with her now-husband for one month when she emailed me that she was pregnant! At the time of this writing, she has a healthy one-year-old. She is happier than ever and is starting a new business with her husband. Everything lined up for her because she was willing to take a leap and do what was right for her despite it looking a little crazy to the outside world. I'm so proud of her for being able to realize that as painful as it was initially, the miscarriage did have a purpose, and what she learned from it changed her entire life for the better.

Leah

Leah came across one of my articles on the Chopra Center website. She had been to fertility specialists but wasn't feeling in her heart that that was the way she wanted to go. Being open to energy work and manifesting, she decided to give this work a try.

External Factors

Leah was in a pretty stressful job at a magazine while working on her doctorate. Deadlines on huge projects left little time for her to get her research and papers done. She had zero time to just breathe. In addition, her husband lived on the other side of the world, so coordinating ovulation involved a lot of planning—which created a lot of expectations and pressure on themselves and each other. Plus they were looking for a house and were not finding any ideal options. There was just too much going on.

Beliefs

Many times the beliefs we are plugging into aren't even ours. They are society's, our doctors', or our family members' beliefs that we have made our own unbeknownst to us. For Leah, the culture her husband's family is from thinks you are an old maid if you don't have a kid by age twenty-seven. They constantly berated her to her face and showed no sensitivity for her situation, so she began to feel more incapable with each encounter.

Leah was also worried deep down that she'd pass on some "bad" family traits to her child. There has been a lot of emotional wounding throughout her family line and there are some recessive physical traits in her family that have "caused" damage to subsequent generations, and she wasn't sure if she should pass that along.

She further worried that her body wasn't strong enough to carry a baby, so her brain—in an attempt to keep her alive—put the kibosh on even getting pregnant so she wouldn't have to endure the pain and humiliation of not being able to do so. Was it true that her body wasn't strong enough? No. But the fear was so strong that her brain assumed it was, so she stayed in a holding pattern.

Leah was also dealing with a common belief among my clients, which is that she was too old or was running out of time. At thirty-nine, she knew deep down that it was possible for her to have a baby, but it was hard not to plug into society's idea of when it's too late and her doctors' belief that IVF was her only option. (Again, IVF is a fine option; it's just not the route she wanted to take.)

It was vital for Leah to work on releasing hurt and anger toward family members, a feeling of obligation toward work, and fears about her body, age, and what family is/can be. It was draining so much of her energy. She felt noticeably lighter after we worked through each issue, not fully realizing how heavy it had been until it wasn't there anymore.

Physical Conditions

In her twenties, Leah had dealt with a lot of health issues stemming from an autoimmune disorder. She did a lot of work on herself, including using Chinese herbs, changing her diet, doing yoga, etc. On an energetic level, autoimmune disorders have to do with an attacking of the inner self. Your immune system is there to protect you, but sometimes it attacks itself. Sometimes when we are trying to protect ourselves, we hurt ourselves. And that made sense from what Leah had said about her place in her family growing up. As an intellectual and nonconformist, she found it pretty hard growing up in an environment where she really couldn't be herself and was not meeting family expectations and they weren't meeting hers.

So her body just attacked itself from the frustration. But she healed from that and then was faced with the fertility issue. Leah has only one functioning ovary and a blocked fallopian tube, so as you can imagine, the doctors' prognosis was bleak. She also had pretty severe endometriosis, which not only is very painful but can mess with your cycles and make conception harder (from a medical perspective). After a botched IUI, she got a severe pelvic infection, which was so painful, and it seemed like there was no end in sight. It was hard not to give up and to feel that maybe this just wasn't going to happen.

Law of Attraction Issues

Due to her strained family life, Leah was not used to being in touch with her emotions and dreaming big. As an intellectual person, it can be a little difficult to leave your brain and get into your body. Even though she did yoga, it was still hard for her to move past the feeling that things were stacked against her and it would just keep being delay after delay. While this attitude was totally understandable given her circumstances, it wasn't so helpful from a Law of Attraction perspective. If like energy attracts like energy and we keep putting out "another thing has gone wrong, another delay," of course there will be another problem and another delay—that's the energy we are being met with. The Universe hears that we aren't capable and we are expecting there to be a problem. When you're in the midst of painful things, it's so hard to just hope or trust that they're going to get better. So sometimes we need to not worry about "fixing" ourselves. From a Law of Attraction perspective, if I believe that I need to "fix" myself, I am repeatedly putting out to the Universe, "I'm broken, I'm broken, I'm not capable, I'm broken." Whereas, if you focus on what is going right, on what you'd love to see (versus what you're scared will happen), then you are energetically aligned with things going right. The Law of Attraction doesn't take a day off. It's always a match to where your energy is and what you're putting out there. So by shifting into what's going right, even if it's small things to start, you can incrementally move your energy over to being able to receive what you actually want.

Sometimes changing our patterns and our environment can go a long way toward shaking up stagnant energy. In one of our sessions, it came up that Leah's husband was going to be on location for a project in a country that she really liked, but she wasn't sure if she should go because of obligations at home. It was a big leap, but she'd be with her husband for a more concentrated period of time and she could do her doctoral research and feel she was making some headway in her life. In our energy session it came up that within three months of her moving there, she would be pregnant. And *bam!* Three months later, she was pregnant. Taking time and space for yourself to expand, heal, and reprioritize is so important. I'm so proud of Leah and her little family.

Kim

External Factors

Kim was in the US on a work visa. Her job was really draining and she had a three-hour round-trip commute every day! She wasn't in a job she loved, but with her visa status she couldn't have a lapse in employment. The stress was getting to her. It was tripping her fight-or-flight response and shutting down her uterus.

Beliefs

Kim had many beliefs operating in the background, some of which were hers. After years of trying, her sense of capability was all but gone. Beliefs like "I'll never be pregnant," "It should have happened already," and "I *need* this to work" were prevalent. She was also dealing with her family's cultural beliefs and judgments as well as financial concerns. So she couldn't help but plug into and be stressed about what family members were saying and their expectations of her. Things just seemed hopeless after such a long journey, but after working through these damaging thoughts, she was able to release her fear and become empowered.

Physical Conditions

Kim was fairly healthy overall, but after trying for seven years, she and her husband had decided to try three rounds of IUI and then IVF. Two failed rounds left her devastated, with no faith in herself or her body. She'd already begun another round when we started working together, and she was full of fear about it not working. After working through these beliefs and fears, she had the same procedure done that she'd had for the other two rounds, but this time it worked! If she hadn't cleaned up her fears and patterns, she would have experienced the same result as the last two. When your body is in so much fear and is stressed-out from work and family dynamics, your fight-or-flight response is triggered. Your brain is worried about self-preservation, and when it feels you can't take care of yourself, it blocks any chance of you creating something that's going to cause you to sacrifice yourself even more. Kim had to learn to claim her space, nourish herself, thank her body for what it was doing, and decide that she could do this. Once she did, her body relaxed enough for her to be pregnant.

All seemed to be great until her husband's mother died. She had been the source of a bit of Kim's stress, but Kim was of course sad for her husband. He had to travel out of the country for the funeral, but she was newly pregnant and couldn't accompany him. She was so stressed about her husband leaving the country and feeling she wasn't a priority on top of grieving the death of her mother-in-law that it was just all too much and her body had to release the baby. Her brain felt she was in emotional overload, and what's one thing that could be taken off her plate? Of course she wanted the baby, but this was one of her life lessons, and though difficult, she needed to explore the reason why something like this would happen. There's always a reason. For her, it was about laying out what she would and would not accept from her partner and family, claiming space, not wasting energy on people who stressed her out, changing jobs (long commute and stressful workload), and allowing herself to heal. She knew she could get pregnant now, and three months later she was pregnant with her little munchkin. At the time of this writing, she has given birth to a beautiful baby boy! The body takes direct orders from the brain. So once she cleared up her thoughts, her body responded with a viable pregnancy.

Law of Attraction Issues

When we first began working together, Kim was emotionally drained and distressed. There was a pervasive cloud of negativity and sadness that she couldn't see her way out of. As many of you can understand, it's not enough to know that it's not helpful to think these negative thoughts. If that's all it took, we'd all be thinking positive all the time. The bottom line, though, is that Kim's energy was continually emitting "This will never work, it hasn't worked yet so it never will, my body is failing me, my mother is driving me nuts, my in-laws are stressing me out, this is hopeless, I can't take anymore." Since like energy attracts like energy, this was a problem. But when you're feeling hopeless, you can't authentically jump to "Everything is just peachy keen."

We did a bunch of emotional work and then started doing some exercises to incrementally move Kim in a more positive direction, including keeping a gratitude journal (being grateful for things you already have opens you up to receiving more things to be grateful for), writing a thank-you letter to her body for what it *does* do, compiling a list of things that were going right in her life, feeling into what she was excited about, and making a victory list to remind her brain that she'd manifested things in the past and could do so again.

Remember that the Universe doesn't hear "I *don't* want ____." It hears what you're focusing on. It's human nature to focus on what's going wrong versus what's going right, but if we expect things to change, we need to start rewiring our brain to expect that positive things are possible. Little by little, Kim migrated over to a more empowered, positive state, and that's when she was able to conceive. The important thing to remember is that this is a work in progress. You have to be patient with yourself. It's like learning a new language, and it takes time to become adept at moving yourself through it.

Conclusion

The infertility journey can seem long, hopeless, and out of our control. Between friends, family, doctors, and society telling us the odds are slim to none that we will get pregnant, let alone have a healthy baby, it feels almost impossible to have confidence in our capability. We rebel against our body for not doing what we think it should, and we push and force out of fear, only to keep going around in circles.

Typical fertility treatments look only at the uterus. But you're not a uterus with feet. You're a person who has relationships, a career, past experiences, etc., that all inform who you are. Most of us aren't taught the skills to fully process these issues, so things get stored in our bodies for years.

It's so painful to think that the thing we want most in the world might be out of reach and we can't control it. But the great news is that you can take some power back in this situation. For some of you, it'll be hard to consider anything other than medical or nutritional intervention, and that's okay! But looking at the whole picture—external factors, beliefs, physical conditions, and where you're putting your energy—can make *the* difference. Some of these things may not seem directly related to your fertility, but I promise you they are. The things outlined in this book are action steps you can take to empower yourself on this journey. Here are some of my previous clients' questions about entering into this kind of work.

Q: There's no guarantee that I'll become pregnant with your technique, so why should I consider this approach?

A: Well, first I would say you're absolutely right: there's no guarantee. I'm not sure what is guaranteed in this life, other than death and taxes, as they say. But if you want to look at the odds, the average IUI success rate is 8 to 20 percent, the IVF success rate is 25 to 50 percent, and my current success rate with my private clients is 66 percent. Not only is the success rate with my approach higher, but it's also not at *all* physically invasive.

Q: Isn't it costly and time-consuming to do this type of approach first?

A: You'd be surprised at how inexpensive it is, considering the alternatives. IUI can be about $1,200 per round, with multiple rounds expected, costing on average $4,800, and IVF can range from $15,000 to $20,000 per round. Many people go through more than one round of this as well, costing upward of $40,000. Working with me costs a fraction of that. Besides the financial costs, we also want to look at the physical and emotional costs of invasive treatments and a prolonged, agonizing journey of feeling like you're trying everything and nothing is working. As you read earlier in the book, there's always an emotional cause to the physical problem, so the sooner we deal with that, the sooner you can move through the situation. So these concepts and techniques are anything *but* time-consuming or a waste of time. They're actually what will clear up this problem for good, and their effects will ripple out to every other area of your life.

Q: You say you do energy work with your clients. What does that mean? Is it a religion? How does it help? How can you do it over the phone?

A: I use distance reiki to clear and shift your energy. It has nothing to do with religion, and there's no dogma you must subscribe to to receive the benefit. The only requirement is that you're open to healing yourself.

Clients report feeling warmth, tingling, twitching, and deep relaxation. As I am doing this work, I am receiving intuitive "hits" in each area. These are seemingly inane visuals with feelings attached to them that let me know what's going on subconsciously with the person—from beliefs they're carrying or traumas they thought they'd dealt with to behavior or external factors that need to shift. From there, we employ the mindset coaching—we speak about what I picked up, where it resonates for you, and how we move forward.

Q: So do you fix the problem with the energy work and then I get better?

A: Um, no. This is not a situation where I wave a magic wand and you're cured. This is a highly cooperative process, and your participation in it is paramount. There is homework for you to do in between sessions that is key in moving forward. It is also of the utmost importance that you be willing to delve into issues you thought you'd already dealt with, as well as be open to releasing what's no longer serving you. I often liken the situation to this: In front of my client there are two doors, Door A and Door B. She wants to go through Door A, so I show her the door, give her the tools to go through it, open the door, and tell her to go ahead. But she bangs her head on Door B. Repeatedly. So I can do energy work and mindset coaching up the wazoo, but it's ultimately up to you to decide to walk through the door. A lot of people don't want that responsibility, but the ones who crack this are the ones who are empowered by the idea that they have the power to shift their situation.

Q: All of this sounds a bit "New Agey." How does mindset end up affecting the body? I don't understand how that could work. Is there any research to back up your findings?

A: Various cultures and practices, from Traditional Chinese Medicine and Ayurvedic medicine to Edgar Cayce, Louise Hay, and Dr. Daniel Amen, have documented the correlation between the mind and its effect on the body. There is also what's known as the Law of Psychophysical Response, which states that for every thought there is a correlating physical reaction. If we're having stressful thoughts, our body has a stressful reaction. This can include slowing down the endocrine and reproductive systems. But evidence shows that when these thoughts are replaced with positivity and relief, the body relaxes and resumes normal functioning because it's no longer in fight-or-flight mode.

An Israeli study led by Professor Eliahu Levitas and presented at a 2004 European Society of Human Reproduction and Embryology conference in Berlin concluded that the success rate of fertility treatments doubled when the women were exposed to mindfulness, meditation, and hypnosis (see http://news.bbc.co.uk/2/hi/health/3849727.stm). Dr. Alice Domar in the US published a research study in 2011 that found that among the women in the study who were previously "infertile" and used a mind-body approach, 55 percent of them were able to conceive naturally (see "Impact of a Group Mind/Body Intervention on Pregnancy Rates in IVF Patients," www.ncbi.nlm.nih.gov/pubmed/21496800). And I've seen it in my practice, where 66 percent of my clients are conceiving naturally by shifting their energy and mindset. It's a matter of stepping aside from the fears and beliefs that haven't been serving you and deciding that you can do this. I am wowed every day in my practice seeing women uncover and move through their blocks and be rewarded with their own little munchkin. There's no dogma you have to believe. This isn't a religion. It's about you being open to releasing what no longer serves you, and knowing that you can do this. Despite there being an energy component to this work, my clients will tell you that I approach it from a pretty practical standpoint and everything has a reason and an application.

Q: What's the benefit of working with a mentor?

A: It took me a long time to realize that I can't do everything myself. As long as I've been in this holistic field, you'd think I'd be able to see all of my own sh—…er…blocks. But we can't see our own stuff. I have a mentor who keeps me on track as well. You, through no fault of your own, are in the middle of your own stuff, so you need an outside perspective. But not just anyone. Someone who has the training to work with numerous types of infertility as well as guide you to work through the mental/emotional causes of it. Even if it's hard for you to wrap your head around that concept right now, if you've tried everything to fix the problem that's keeping you up at night and it isn't working, don't you owe it to yourself to try?

Q: I don't have time—I'm too busy.

A: Aren't we all? I've been there. That's the great thing about the phone sessions. We work around your schedule and you don't have to *go* anywhere. There's no worrying about traffic, parking, or making it home on time. It's done on an agreed schedule based on your availability. If you're saying you don't have enough time, chances are it means you're not making enough time for *yourself*. And that needs to change. As you read earlier in the book, if your brain thinks you're spread too thin, it doesn't want to add another thing for you to take care of. Believe it or not, your busy schedule is contributing to the ailment that brought you to me in the first place. You *deserve* this little munchkin. So make time for yourself.

Q: I can't afford it.

A: Listen, this one I can empathize with. I know that in this economy it's tough to feel like you're throwing money toward something that's not a "necessity." I get it. It's not food, clothing, or rent. But I have to tell you that where you are is a reflection of what's going on inside. We have no problem spending money to buy clothes and gadgets we don't need to fill some void we can't pinpoint. We spend money on fertility treatments like IUI, which even with insurance can be $400 to $1,200 per round, and IVF, which can be $15,000 to $20,000 per round, not to mention therapy, physical therapy, hormone treatments, pain medications, and the list goes on. And they all treat symptoms. We need to get to the cause—the root. And I can help you do that. Can you put a price on naturally conceiving the baby you *thought* you *couldn't* have? (And trust me, this is a hell of a lot cheaper than fertility treatments!) Once you achieve this, the benefits will ripple out exponentially to all areas of your life. See the Results page at www.FusionFertility.com to read stories of people who have been through it and got better results than they could imagine. You can do this and I am so excited to help guide you.

Q: I've done everything to get pregnant. Why would this approach work?

A: I would bet that the other approaches you've tried have not involved looking at your beliefs and mindset. As we've discussed throughout this book, what you're believing and where you're putting your energy matter. Your outcome is directly related to how you approach the situation. Many times we take on the beliefs of doctors, family, and society that we are too old and are running out of time, etc., or even our own beliefs that we should be pregnant by now, or that getting pregnant is hard. And when this "app" is running in the background, it's diverting so much energy from you moving forward toward what you want. So none of these methods will work until your mindset shifts. Most of the world isn't aware that mindset is a factor in fertility, and even fewer know how to address it. Once you shift these things, the benefits ripple out to every area of your life and open your energy and your body to receiving what you want.

If you feel like you want some individualized attention as part of the next step in your journey, you can visit www.FusionFertility.com to find out about my programs. I work with my private clients to clear their energy, uncover blocks, hold them accountable for patterns, and support them like nobody's business to help them achieve what they're wanting most.

This approach would be helpful for you if you

- are tired of the frustration and disappointment.

- know something needs to shift but don't know what.

- are thinking about medical intervention, but the cost is too great or you secretly feel like you can do it on your own.

- have tried medical intervention, like IUI and IVF, and it didn't work, but you aren't willing to give up.

- know you're meant to be a mom no matter what.

- understand that there's a mindset component involved and want to learn how to harness it to have the pregnancy you deserve.

- are willing to do the emotional work necessary, especially when it gets uncomfortable.

You have more control in this process than you've been led to believe. And I'd love to help you on your way to conceiving naturally on your terms.

In the meantime, *brava* for taking an energetic step toward what you deserve! Take what you can from this book to make some shifts. There are so many things you can do to move yourself forward, and this gives you a good place to start.

I wish you all the best on your journey. *Know* that you can do this, mama.

Recommended Reading

★ Visit my website, www.FusionFertility.com, and register to receive your **free Conceivable Tool Kit**.

Dyer, Wayne. *The Power of Intention*. Carlsbad, CA: Hay House, 2005.

Hay, Louise. *You Can Heal Your Life*. Carlsbad, CA: Hay House, 1984.

Hicks, Esther, and Jerry Hicks. *The Amazing Power of Deliberate Intent*. Carlsbad, CA: Hay House, 2006.

————. *Ask and It Is Given*. Carlsbad, CA: Hay House, 2006.

————. *Money and the Law of Attraction*. Carlsbad, CA: Hay House, 2008.

Katie, Byron. *Loving What Is*. New York: Three Rivers, 2003.

Lipton, Bruce H. *The Biology of Belief*. Carlsbad, CA: Hay House, 2004.

Rankin, Lissa, MD. *Mind Over Medicine*. Carlsbad, CA: Hay House, 2013.

Rose, Evette. *Metaphysical Anatomy*. Create Space, 2013.

Steele, Cassie Premo. *Moon Days*. Summerhouse Press, 1999.

Tolle, Eckhart. *A New Earth*. New York: Penguin, 2005.

Weed, Susun. *Down There: Sexual and Reproductive Health the Wise Woman Way*. Woodstock, NY: Ash Tree Publishing, 2011.

————. *Wise Woman Herbal for the Childbearing Year.* Woodstock, NY: Ash Tree Publishing, 1986.

To Ease Fear Around Natural Childbirth

Gaskin, Ina May. *Ina May's Guide to Breastfeeding.* New York: Bantam Books, 2009.

————. *Ina May's Guide to Childbirth.* New York: Bantam Books, 2003.

Mongan, Marie. *HypnoBirthing: The Mongan Method.* Deerfield Beach, FL: Health Communications, 2005.

The Business of Being Born DVD. Barranca Productions. Burbank, CA: New Line Home Entertainment, 2008.

More Business of Being Born DVD. 2011.

Acknowledgments

It was never my intention to write a book. It organically grew out of my work with my clients and classes that I've taught. Life is such a curly-Q trajectory; sometimes I can't believe how lucky I am that I get to do this for a living. I certainly wouldn't be able to it without some special people.

To my husband, Joe: Thank you for believing in me even when I didn't, for being my biggest fan, and for your support through thick and thin. I love you.

To my parents: For always supporting whatever crazy idea I had. I lucked out in the supportive parents department and I can't thank you enough. It's given me courage many times in my life, and I am forever grateful.

To my sister-in-law Sherri: For being my first fertility client, for being brave enough to go on this journey, and for truly changing my life. It gives me such joy to see you and my brother with your little munchkin and I'm so proud of you and thankful for you.

To my friend of almost twenty years and business mentor, Stephanie McWilliams: I seriously don't know where I'd be without you. Thank you for helping me work through my limiting beliefs and showing me that I could make a living doing what I am on the planet to do. I can never repay you for your guidance not only in business but in how I see the world.

To my agent Tina: I never thought I'd find a fellow Reiki Master as an agent! Thank you for taking a chance on my little book and on me! Thank you for tirelessly working to find me the right publisher for this book that's going to help so many women.

Thanks to all of the folks at Llewellyn Worldwide, especially my editor Amy Glaser for recognizing the potential and helping me get this book to the women who need it.

Index

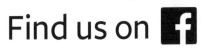 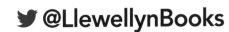